TRUSTING ON THE EDGE

Managing uncertainty and vulnerability in the midst of serious mental health problems

Patrick Brown and Michael Calnan

First published in Great Britain in 2012 by

The Policy Press
University of Bristol
Fourth Floor
Beacon House
Queen's Road
Bristol BS8 1QU
UK
Tel +44 (0)117 331 4054
Fax +44 (0)117 331 4093
e-mail tpp-info@bristol.ac.uk
www.policypress.co.uk

North American office:

The Policy Press
c/o The University of Chicago Press
1427 East 60th Street
Chicago, IL 60637, USA
t: +1 773 702 7700
f: +1 773-702-9756
e:sales@press.uchicago.edu
www.press.uchicago.edu

British Library Cataloguing in Publication Data
A catalogue record for this book is available from the British Library.

Library of Congress Cataloging-in-Publication Data
A catalog record for this book has been requested.

ISBN 978 1 84742 889 9 hardcover

Cover design by Robin Hawes
Front cover: image kindly supplied by www.istockphoto.com
Printed and bound by CPI Group (UK) Ltd, Croydon, CR0 4YY
The Policy Press uses environmentally responsible print partners

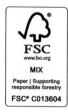

FSC
www.fsc.org
MIX
Paper | Supporting
responsible forestry
FSC® C013604

Contents

Preface

> We delegate certain things to other people, not merely because we cannot do them, but because we do not wish to run the risk of error.... For each occupation that one studies one should, I believe, seek to determine just what it is that is delegated to the persons in the occupation and what are the attitudes and feelings involved on both sides. (Cherrington-Hughes, 1994: 81–2)

The need to delegate certain responsibilities to others and a corresponding reliance upon these others is a basic feature of the social, economic and political worlds. Whether we are depending upon a close friend, trading based on certain expectations or casting a vote for a particular candidate, notions of trust are vital in facilitating this process of delegation and the peace of mind we have in doing so. Lately, both academics and the mass media have been concerned with the apparent difficulty in trusting within late-modern society and the implications of this threatened or 'declining' trust for social capital, economic trade and political authority. At the centre of these concerns is the suggestion that trust is something both vital and endangered.

The complex manifestations of trust within political systems, or financial markets, are well beyond the scope of this study; instead, this book seeks to shed light on trust within the social context of healthcare. Nonetheless, while trust relations are in some senses very much context-specific, an examination of trust within one case of delegation can surely be instructive for understandings of how trust functions in other settings. In particular, we hope that by examining trust where it is particularly vital, and particularly endangered, the analysis expressed in this volume may say something about trust that is pertinent beyond the delegation of care for people experiencing serious mental health problems. Of course, we also seek to make a contribution to comprehension of the nature of trust, the factors behind it and the ramifications of its presence or absence in this important healthcare and social policy setting.

People experiencing psychosis do not necessarily choose to have their care delegated to mental health professionals themselves, and yet in many senses they may trust (or distrust, or mistrust) nevertheless. This issue of trust and its relation to (free) choice, as developed in Chapter Four, is important within a number of different environments (social, economic and political). In a certain sense, bound up with this issue of whether vulnerable people have significant choice or not, many have questioned whether trust is a rational approach within a specific situation, given that we never really know what the trustee will do and because there is always the chance that we might be let down; this concern with rationality is pursued in Chapter Three.

—

That people seek to rely upon others as a means for overcoming the 'risk of error', as suggested in the earlier quote, has important implications for our understanding of the role of trust and, accordingly, how delegated individuals and organisations function – in seeking to avert risk and, correspondingly, blame. The experiences of delegated individuals (mental health professionals in our case study) and, in turn, how these actors function within delegated organisations is explored in Chapter Five. In Chapter Two, meanwhile, we explore trust from the perspective of the person in need – paying particular attention to the relative import of the individual or the delegated organisation of which the individual professional is a part. Along with Chapter One, Chapter Two also considers the very nature of trust and how trust (and, correspondingly, delegation) is possible even when individuals' past experiences might warrant otherwise. These reflections suggest that trust is perhaps not as endangered as some might fear, but nonetheless we argue in Chapter Six that social settings (especially healthcare organisations) which work to enhance levels of trust are more likely to be effective and efficient in assisting vulnerable individuals in need.

The book is a means of dealing with these more general, theoretical questions around trust while at the same time seeking to ground the discussion in a distinct empirical context of how service users, and those delegated the role of helping them (by society if not always by the service users), manage their experiences of uncertainty and vulnerability through trust or alternative approaches. We are very much indebted to the generous professionals and managers who were so keen to cooperate with this research. We do not name them here for anonymity reasons, but we would in any case like to express our warm thanks.

Similarly the service users who gave up their time and shared their experiences were vital to us being able to write about trust in a format that is (we hope) meaningfully connected to the reality of day-to-day experiences and thus take the subject matter of this book beyond mere theoretical conjecture. We do not name these service users, again to honour the anonymity that was promised them. Instead, we use numbers so that readers can straightforwardly make linkages between views expressed in different parts of the text. We use pseudonyms in certain boxes when particular individuals are written about at greater length so as to separate these contextual references from others in the book – once more to assist in preserving these participants' anonymity. The research was made possible by a grant from the Economic and Social Research Council.

We have both contributed to the research and the writing of the book and share responsibility for its contents. Patrick took the lead in writing the Introduction and Chapters One to Five, while Michael took the lead over Chapter Six. We would both like to thank a number of colleagues who have provided much useful information, insight, advice and feedback. We have presented several papers related to the contents of the book at various conferences and workshops and received a lot of useful input from these. Patrick is grateful to a number of colleagues at the University of Amsterdam for their constructive comments, while Paul Langthorne and Richard Brown have offered many valuable insights on the topics covered in the book. He also learned a lot from being involved in the 'Trust and Health' workshop hosted by the Bioethics Research Group at NTNU, Trondheim and would like to thank Marit Solbjør and her colleagues for inviting him. Michael extends his thanks to those at the University of Sydney and University of Tasmania who engaged with various aspects of the arguments presented here during his sabbatical time in Australia. Amanda Scrivener and George Szmukler are two senior practitioners who have assisted us as we have sought to write something relevant to a mental healthcare audience. However, the authors alone are responsible for any deficiencies within the following chapters.

Risk and trust in late-modern society

The study of trust presented in this book is predominantly theoretical in nature, though our analyses of the concept are nevertheless grounded in, and illustrated through, qualitative data collected in our research within community-based services that deliver healthcare for people experiencing serious mental health problems – especially those with diagnoses of psychosis – in Southern England. The empirical research that informs the theoretical frameworks we develop not only serves to enable more robust, empirically relevant conceptualisations, but also allows us to consider the relevance of trust where it is most vital and yet potentially most problematic – amidst especially heightened levels of vulnerability and uncertainty. Thus, our research in these settings was in part motivated by the potential utility of emerging insights for mental health services, but furthermore because this setting represents a *crucible* of conditions pertinent to informing our understandings of the concept of trust. Correspondingly, this book is intended as both an extension of social theories of trust, while simultaneously offering more practical insights into the relevance and functioning of trust within mental healthcare and other services seeking to meet the needs of vulnerable people.

Following understandings of theory development as an extension out of careful exploration of cases (Burawoy, 1998), and in relating the micro to the macro through 'forensic analysis' (Inglis, 2010), our account of trust takes place at the level of social theory, pertaining to more generally occurring social processes, yet this analysis is very much informed through the 'clues, episodes and events' of a micro-investigation of social relations in a particular context. As touched upon already, and as we will go on to argue later in this Introduction and in following chapters, there are many features of the social experiences and relations visible in our data that render this research context pertinent to understandings of trust in late-modern societies at the more general and even macro-level. In this sense, our presentation of trust is very relevant to considerations of broader dynamics occurring across many late-modern welfare states in the global North.

Late-modernity and the illumination of uncertainties

The concept of *late-modernity* that is being invoked here is one pertaining chiefly to 'crisis'. While Habermas (1976: 1) makes this connection with particular regard to political institutions, economic and welfare management, and legitimacy, the 'lateness' or destabilising of modernity can be conceptualised as a much broader phenomenon. In this sense, many of the central tenets of the project of modernity – scientific knowledge, its deployment by experts as incentivised by state institutions, and the enfranchisement of the masses to participate in the benefits and hopes of the Enlightenment – are increasingly subject to circumspection, contestation and cynicism. A heightened awareness of, and sensitivity towards, the manifold dysfunctional consequences of this 'Age of Reason' (Weber, 1968; Beck, 1992; Porter, 2001) have led to many notions that had previously remained at the level of 'taken-for-grantedness' – such as the *emancipatory* project of science or the aptitude of scientists and medical experts – being called increasingly into question (Beck, 1992).

The undermining of these bastions of *modern* society has a number of ramifications for how institutions and individuals negotiate decision-making and planning in respect to the short, medium and longer terms. As many background assumptions, norms and values are opened to scrutiny and doubt, it follows that a number of costs are borne by decision-makers (organisations or individuals) due to the difficulties in coping with these emerging uncertainties:

> It is only under the pressure of approaching problems that relevant components of such background knowledge are torn out of their unquestioned familiarity and brought to consciousness as something in need of being ascertained. It takes an earthquake to make us aware that we had regarded the ground on which we stand everyday as unshakable. (Habermas, 1984: 400)

Although it is important not to exaggerate conceptions of 'late'-ness, as if at one point all was considered knowable and stable whereas now all is fluid, the range of uncertainties that have to be negotiated have been described as a growing feature of a more mobile, function-differentiated and globalised world; one where interactions with strangers, abstract systems and alternative conceptions are a growing part of the everyday experiences of a rising number of people (Giddens, 1990, 1991).

Formats of explanation for this illuminating of uncertainty within recent times are wide-ranging – varying across epistemological perspectives and levels of analysis. Grand narratives note: the self-defeating tendencies within governing institutions due to the way these respond to economic difficulties, with corresponding ramifications for the socio-cultural sphere (Habermas, 1976); the expansion of a certain form of liberal-capitalism and the changes it renders to trajectories/experiences of work, poverty and class alongside associated distancing of relations in terms of time and space (Bauman, 2000); and the associated individualisation (imperatives placed on contingencies of individuals' decisions) amidst the breakdown of institutions and other tools by which actors make sense of the world (Giddens, 1991; Beck, 1992), combined with a heightening awareness (established through science and disseminated by the mass media) that scientific developments pose an array of environmental and health risks – the effects of which are keenly contested (Beck, 1992). Other approaches (eg Furedi, 2002) have connected such macro-perspectives with more mid-level analyses relating to cultural processes and the media–driven construction of social problems (Best, 1999; Cohen, 2002).

Arguably, one of the most incisive approaches has been that of Wilkinson (2010: 27–34), who develops Weber's concern with theodicy and the problem of suffering to connect fundamental changes in society with more micro–level manifestations of risk–based approaches. Understanding the project of modernity as one intended to reduce suffering helps explain the development of contradictory processes whereby religion is displaced by science and yet increasingly sophisticated understandings of the natural world render heightened levels of dissatisfaction (as reductions in suffering are not achieved). A fundamental tension accordingly emerges between rational/evidence–based interventions designed to alleviate social problems and the requirement of governing institutions to attend to the 'charismatic' (in the Weberian sense) needs of citizens as suffering endures (Wilkinson, 2010).

These understandings of tension, contradiction and crisis are applicable and clearly visible within healthcare systems as well as welfare states more generally. Taylor–Gooby (2000: 3) describes the 'timid prosperity' encountered within many welfare states and health services whereby standards of living and a vast range of health indicators suggest improving outcomes and yet 'peoples' opinions and perceptions of the NHS have not only not improved, they have worsened' (Appleby and Alvarez–Rosete, 2003: 29). In England and Wales, tendencies towards a more systematic, evidence–based and efficient healthcare provision have yielded significant advances in biomedical outcomes, yet these advances would seem to result in a more commodified form of health provision (Harrison, 2009), which is ineffective at meeting the 'charismatic' and holistic needs of patients (Harrison and Smith, 2004).

Concurrently, the more 'consumerist' approach adopted by a number of patients, combined with the contingently empowering phenomena of the internet (see Nettleton et al, 2005) and the broader dissemination of biomedical knowledge, entails that many NHS professionals are faced with increasing challenges in providing what they deem as appropriate care while maintaining legitimacy in the eyes of these *clients* (Newman and Vidler, 2006). Such a challenging of medical expertise (Hardey, 1999), and a tentative venture back towards medical pluralism (Wade et al, 2008), makes plain that it is not simply the major ruling institutions that are in a state of crisis; healthcare systems, biomedicine and professionalism are all confronted by a more glaring uncertainty.

Strategies of managing vulnerability in the face of uncertainty: risk and trust

Difficulties and strategies of decision-making

The illumination of the myriad uncertainties faced by social actors, or alternatively the apparent erosion of existing mechanisms for managing a range of unknowables, renders many individuals more prone to experiences of vulnerability and anxiety (Wilkinson, 2001). Late-modern social processes leave actors more individualised (for a critical reading, see Elliott, 2002) – with individuals held more responsible for outcomes contingent on their personal choices – yet the information on which these agents may draw to inform these choices is more readily acknowledged as problematic and fallible. Furthermore, the range of sources of knowledge available, their technical sophistication and the breadth of paradigms via which knowledge can be considered, all combine to represent a significant level of decision-making complexity. Finally, the sources of these multiple arrays of information are increasingly tending to be consolidated within abstract systems (Giddens, 1990), with the decision-maker often separated from the 'source' of knowledge by both space and time (Giddens, 1990). These abstract systems in the late-modern era tend to necessitate the dependency of the individual on an array of 'absent others' (Giddens, 1994) with whom one has little or no interaction.

Combined, these issues of uncertainty, complexity and abstractness (as encountered by individuals who are vulnerable – not least to the contingent outcomes of a poor decision) have led to a large growth in social theoretical considerations that attempt to disentangle and analyse a range of challenges to the individual decision-maker. Many of these empirical and theoretical foci, which have become increasingly prominent within sociological discussions, can be loosely bracketed under the heading 'modes by which actors (individuals, groups and organisations) seek to manage vulnerability in the context of this uncertainty'.

On the subject of decision-making by individuals in everyday life, Zinn (2008a) develops a typology of different formats for determining appropriate action amidst uncertainty. These alternatives are arranged along a spectrum from the rational, via the 'between rational', towards the non-rational. Approaches that may be considered 'rational' within a number of social-scientific paradigms are those that entail aspects of calculation (of probability and consequences – ie *risk*), and which thus enable techniques for dealing with negative outcomes through insurance or provision. Those that might be deemed from certain perspectives as 'non-rational' include belief, faith and hope, as these modes are only able to 'manage' negative outcomes through avoidance or endurance. This topic of the 'rational' and 'non-rational' will receive much more critical attention in the early parts of Chapter Three.

Zinn's most interesting contribution is in describing a number of strategies that he posits as 'in between' the rational and the non-rational. This category includes trust, intuition and emotion and, following Gigerenzer (2007), Zinn relates these approaches to a growing research corpus pertaining to *heuristics* and other such 'pre-rational' short cuts to information processing that are intrinsic to everyday decisions. These considerations of how individuals, through modes of decision-making that are both calculative and less-than-calculative, are able to act in the midst of uncertainty connect with a vast corpus of judgement and decision-making psychology (following Tversky and Kahneman, 1974) and related discussions within economics, particularly through the work of Simon (eg 1982).

—

It is *individuals*, especially those whose actions are embedded within processes of trust and distrust, who are of particular concern to our study. However, the setting of our research, as is the case with many actions within late-modernity, involves these actors interfacing with *institutions* (in our case mental health services). Simon's (1982) work, of course, also relates to decisions taken within organisations, and it is the nexus between individuals (especially service users, professionals and managers) and the institutions they relate to that will emerge as vital to understandings of trust within the following chapters. Institutions, particularly vast organisations such as the NHS, exhibit different tendencies in terms of their decision-making to those of individuals – especially with regard to the types of decisions that appear in Zinn's non-rational and 'in between' categories.

In a similar mode to Zinn's spectrum, analyses of organisational decisions amidst uncertainty have over a number of decades conceptualised approaches as more or less calculative in nature. Fully 'rational'-calculative approaches have for a long time been recognised as impossible for organisations to achieve (Lindblom, 1959). Much research in this area has instead asked questions regarding the extent to which calculative approaches are desirable – assessing the impact of varying formats for managing transactions (between individuals within organisations, or between organisations) within uncertain conditions and their impact on a range of outcomes. Transaction cost economics, significantly influenced by the work of Williamson (eg 1975), has developed a number of innovative analyses in this vein, a range of which are relatively compatible with sociological approaches to organisations and will be returned to later.

Risk, calculative decision-making and its application in the NHS

The concept of risk – a vital one for our study – emerged as a key concept within the social-scientific literature, particularly economics, as a means to describe the more calculative approaches to uncertainty that were able to be applied by firms in particular conditions. Knight (1921; see also Langlois and Cosgel, 1993: 460) differentiates between approaches to uncertainty that: seek to categorise and probabilistically calculate in their response to uncertainty ('calculable' risk); distinguish between potential outcomes in the face of uncertainty, but where numeric calculation of their likelihood is seen as impossible (categorisable uncertainty); and recognise uncertainty in a more vague and nebulous manner. Socially constructed assumptions (Schutz, 1972) within prevailing organisational systems (Japp and Kusche, 2008) can be seen as influencing the chosen configurations of these various approaches, and thus the applications of knowledge forms within each system (Brown and Calnan, forthcoming).

Risk approaches have become an increasingly common approach within modernity as techniques for estimating probability and planning for consequences have become more sophisticated, but also, from a more cultural perspective, due to an increasing preoccupation with considerations around 'the calculability of consequences' (Weber, 1978: 351) across various domains within society. This correlated existence of technological possibilities on the one hand, and cultural beliefs and processes on the other, is at the heart of social-scientific accounts of risk – with some beginning with the former and the *advent* of risk technologies as a path to understanding the latter (Beck, 1992), while others (Douglas, 1992) see risk as merely a more recent manifestation of cultural processes and tensions that have long existed within and between groups.

A more in-depth consideration of sociological and anthropological approaches to risk is beyond the scope of this book though are usefully considered within other recent texts (Mythen and Walklate, 2006; Zinn, 2008b; Wilkinson, 2010). Of more pressing interest for the current analysis is the application of risk within healthcare organisations such as the NHS and, furthermore, the particular manifestations of risk management within the approach of English mental health services to the apparent dangers associated with people experiencing mental illness. Once again, we see a sustained and dynamic interaction between the development of bureaucratic and biomedical technologies on the one hand, and political and socio-cultural norms on the other. We will consider these tendencies – the bureaucratic and the biomedical – in sequence.

There are a number of interwoven narratives that are important to understanding the emergence of risk as a key concept within health policy, but there is a general agreement that notions of risk, especially those focused on the individual, are overtaking need as the basis of health policy provision (Kemshall, 2002: 1) – with this especially the case in mental health (Pilgrim, 2007). The tendencies to which Kemshall refers emerged more explicitly and radically within policy proposals in the second half of the 1990s and into the 2000s; however, the development of a comprehensive strategy for governing clinical practice in relation to risk (eg through clinical governance), and the plan to revise the Mental Health Act 1983 first announced in 1998, are best understood as culminations of longer-running currents rather than wholly novel phenomena (Szmukler, 2001; Flynn, 2002; Pilgrim and Rogers, 2009).

Various authors have argued that a number of highly publicised failings in the NHS across the 1990s were significant drivers leading to the determined politicisation of risk management strategies – of clinical practice right across the NHS, and of 'dangerous' people in contact with mental health services (Freedman, 2002; Hallam, 2002). The initial media moral panics in response to clinical failings and heightened morbidity in a leading regional surgical unit (Bristol Royal Infirmary), and the murder of Jonathan Zito by Christopher Clunis who had been in contact with a number of different mental health services, have been seen as watershed moments, which galvanised risk approaches (Smith, 1998; Alaszewski, 2002; Brown, 2006; Warner, 2006). These incidents were followed by further scrutiny after subsequent failings, alongside various formats of inquiries into these failings. These investigations themselves form particular narratives for understanding failure and seeking to pre-empt lapses in the future (Alaszewski, 2002; Kewell, 2006; Warner, 2006; Alaszewski and Brown, 2012).

The move towards the governance of clinical quality (and especially safety) in healthcare has been described as an example of governmentality (Flynn, 2002) due to the manner by which it has involved a profound shift in the way knowledge is to be applied by medical professionals and the consequent impact on how professionals reflect on the 'conduct of their conduct'. Warner (2006) provides an insightful case study in this vein, exploring how a group of mental health professionals, as a result of their awareness of the findings of the Ritchie Report into the care of Christopher Clunis, performed ongoing self-surveillance in light of this knowledge – with their professional practice becoming more defensive as a result.

Alaszewski (2002) describes how clinical governance seeks to move the management of knowledge from an individual dimension into the collective, and from a tacit application towards a more explicit form. In this sense, there has been a general shift from what Lam refers to as 'embodied knowledge', held by the individual in tacit form, to 'encoded knowledge', by which knowledge is disseminated across a community of doctors in the form of explicit guidelines, directives and universalising standards. Flynn (2002: 168) goes on to label this approach one of 'machine bureaucracy', through which there is a high standardisation of knowledge and where individual autonomy is replaced by strong organisational control.

These more bureaucratic forms of risk management across the NHS were preceded by the development of the Care Programme Approach (CPA) in mental health services, through which the interests and safety of mental healthcare patients is to be ensured through ongoing systematic assessment, planning and reviewing of care as coordinated by a particular professional (Department of Health, 1995). The eventual revision of the Mental Health Act 1983 (Department of Health, 2007) was similarly motivated by apparent failings in care, but had quite different emphases – relating to the grounds by which individuals with mental illness can be forcibly detained for treatment (see Pilgrim, 2007). Yet what all three policy directions (clinical governance, CPA and the new mental health law) have in common are aspirations regarding the application and harnessing of technologies of risk management – either more 'new public management'-bureaucratic or more clinical-diagnostic – to provide better, safer and more consistent healthcare.

Inherent within these applications of calculative, risk-oriented approaches within the coordination of healthcare are a range of assumptions about the nature of medicine, mental healthcare and the application of clinical knowledge within these settings. The assumption that healthcare professionals deal with *regular* manifestations of illness to the extent that its presentation, diagnosis and treatment is predictable and amenable to protocols and calculative prediction is highly evident. Moreover, even where complexity and subtlety are acknowledged, it is still taken for granted that sufficiently refined approaches of audit and target frameworks can drive quality and minimise risk (Brown and Calnan, 2011: 20). These assumptions are scrutinised in the next subsection.

The difficulties in managing risk and the potential for trust

A number of authors referred to in the preceding subsection have evaluated these calculative-bureaucratic directions as problematic (eg Szmukler, 2001; Alaszewski, 2002; Flynn, 2002; Pilgrim, 2007). Brown and Calnan (2010) draw some of these overarching considerations together in acknowledging the problems of managing uncertainty through more calculative and bureaucratic formats. Drawing on Sennett (2008) as a conceptual framework, we acknowledge the fallibility of the craftwork of *human* healthcare professionals, but argue that the recent tendencies towards *bureaucratic* solutions are more problematic still. Central to this critique are doubts over the uniformity, predictability and thus calculability of the 'risks' involved, which can be seen as congruent with work on the screening of mental health service users for violence (Szmukler, 2003; Langan, 2010). Returning to the work of Knight (1921) referred to earlier, the phenomena that recent policies seek to approach through bureaucratic stipulation and control are categorisable or merely known levels of uncertainty, but mistaken for 'calculable risks'. Bureaucratic approaches to these phenomena are, by their calculable and generalising paradigms, unable to successfully manage this uncertainty and may be weakening control rather than strengthening it – as regards clinical governance (Brown, 2008a) or the management of 'risky' individuals (Szmukler, 2003).

At a more general and macro-level, a further way of considering the limitations in attempts at control through risk management and bureaucracy emerges within the questions over the nature of social and political order and debates as to how this is achieved, following Hobbes (1968 [1651]). If order is achievable through the effective administration of instrumental forms of sanctions and incentives, then bureaucratic forms are potentially highly effective. However, a whole range of social theorists have argued to the contrary and emphasised, following Durkheim, the 'non-contractual' aspects of social order and the effective processes by which control is exercised and adhered to through prevailing discourses, norms and values (for an overview, see Habermas, 1987: 204–34; for an abridged/schematic version applied to healthcare, see Brown, 2008a). The blindness of bureaucracy to the non-contractual, and its inability to replicate norms and values in a format that is meaningful for human action and decision-making, therefore renders more bureaucratic forms quite impotent to enforce order.

These limitations may be especially true with regard to achieving control of actors existing amidst various uncertain conditions, due to the range of possible behaviours and outcomes that need to be taken into account. Notions of 'space' can be considered relevant here in considering these limitations of bureaucracy. The forms of control/management that are aimed at in terms of clinical risk (clinical governance) or risk assessment (recent mental health policy) are by their very nature systematic, generalised and thus ambivalent to context. The attempts to standardise clinical practice across the NHS, or risk assessment in mental health services, thus represents a highly encoded application of knowledge (Lam, 2000), which, in contrast to more embodied forms (Lam, 2000; Alaszewski, 2002;

Nettleton et al, 2008), is highly distanced from the decision-making context and therefore impoverished in terms of the social, clinical and tacit experiences (and knowledge derived from these) that are vital to effective decisions amidst uncertainty.

Schön (1983) emphasises the artistry required in the successful practice of medicine as opposed to a more technical/rational model. In particular, he highlights the recurrent presence of abnormal situations where usual protocol is not sufficient and creative reflection is necessary. The move to encoded knowledge (Lam, 2000) in recent 'scientific-bureaucratic' (Harrison, 2009) modes of healthcare not only fails to consider that it is these atypical scenarios, where protocol is inadequate, which are also potentially the riskiest, but, in their more everyday application, bureaucratic 'routines tend to become increasingly dysfunctional over time: not only do they fail to adjust to new circumstances but "shortcuts" gradually intrude, some of which only help professionals to cope with pressure at the expense of helping their clients' (Eraut, 1994: 112).

In terms of *space*, bureaucratic management amidst uncertainty thus creates distance between the decision-making apparatus and the problem to be solved. Considerations of *time* are also significant to understandings of the 'risk' approach and its potential limitations in healthcare contexts. Alaszewski and Burgess (2007) describe the gradual change in the nature of risk management in its relation to the aggregation of knowledge regarding the past and the present and its application to the future. These authors chart the development of risk from its highly statistical, prediction-focused roots in the 17th century to a more forensic approach by which the major concern was the causality behind the negative outcomes as much as the likelihood of an event recurring in the future. More recently, it is argued that a 'precautionary principal' is skewing considerations of risk decision-making, by which the fear of *future* institutional failures in managing risk becomes an overriding factor that stifles effectual decision-making in the face of uncertainty:

> The precautionary approach focuses on uncertainty rather than risk, and uncertainty is often an openly posed condition rather than the bounded and specific challenge common to the more technical conception of risk. Neither foresight nor hindsight provide a good guide to risk management and the safest approach is risk aversion. Precaution is not so much a guide to (future) action, as the recommendation that inaction is the safest course in the face of threatening uncertainty. (Alaszewski and Burgess, 2007: 356)

The inherent tendency for risk management within institutions to become preoccupied with minimising 'reputational risk' to the institution ahead of risk management for the good of society (Rothstein, 2006), or patients, underlines the case for alternative approaches to uncertainty such as trust (Brown and Calnan, 2010, 2011). Trust has been recognised as highly significant within healthcare organisations for the way it facilitates healthcare outcomes for patients, as well as its enhancing of efficiency and interactions within organisations (Gilson et al, 2005). Davies and Mannion (2000: 262) suggest that when the nature of agent behaviour is straightforwardly measurable and 'unambiguous', bureaucratic or 'checking' forms of coping with governing clinical practice within healthcare organisations are highly appropriate. In other settings, trust, or at least a balance between trust and checking, is necessary due to the manner by which 'softer information and informal relationships often underpin formal contracts' (Davies and Mannion, 2000: 251).

On a similar basis, Williamson (1993: 479) asserts that 'economic activity will be better organized where there is an appreciation for and intentional use of informal organization' and sees trust as vital for the existence of such an 'atmosphere' of cooperative interaction. Returning to decision-making by distinct *individuals*, rather than at the organisational level, the informal and cultural channels to which Williamson refers are important for actors such as patients and professionals – in enabling them to overcome uncertainty through the exchange of knowledge through open communication (Dew et al, 2007). This is not to say that uncertainty is able to be eradicated, but rather that efficient communication is facilitated via the ability to bracket away various 'unknowns' through assumptions in the competency of others and a compatibility of each other's goals. In turn, more effective communication will enable greater levels of certainty for both the professional (in making diagnoses and interpreting the effectiveness of interventions) and the patient (in understanding the professional's advice and interpretation of their condition).

Proximity and familiarity – which are both enabled by, and products of, trust – are vital for this knowledge to come about (Adler, 2001) and, accordingly, trusting environments can be seen as conducive to the further building of trust relations. In contrast, organisations or settings where there is a deficiency of trust, through the inhibiting of familiarity, mean that trust may be harder to win. It is in this sense that the bureaucratic has been held as negative for trust in that it stifles proximity, obstructs communication and institutionalises checking rather than trusting behaviour (Brown, 2008b). Recent tendencies in health policy can, accordingly, be seen as insensitive or ambivalent to trust (Hood, 2005), or, in Williamson's (1993: 480) terms, the 'neglect of such interaction effects is encouraged by piecemeal calculativeness, which is to say by an insensitivity to atmosphere'.

Atmospheres of trust? Various forms of 'hyphenated' trust

One of the central themes of this study is the question of how, and to what extent, trust is still possible when the 'atmosphere' for trust is far from conducive. The question of the nature of trust in such settings becomes more pertinent still when we take into account very high levels of vulnerability and uncertainty – as may be experienced by people with serious mental health problems and also the professionals who care for them – which make trust both more necessary and less likely (Brown et al, 2009). These direct considerations will be pursued across the six chapters that follow this Introduction. Meanwhile, the remainder of this preliminary chapter will be chiefly concerned with sketching an outline of various institutional dynamics that can be seen as representing 'atmospheres' which are more or less conducive to trust.

In attending to these broader settings, we follow several social-theoretical accounts (eg Luhmann, 1979; Giddens, 1991) that note how trust is essentially a process taking place between individuals but which nonetheless is facilitated by, and embedded within, a range of trust-like norms and assumptions towards broader systems or institutions. This is especially the case when, in late-modern settings, actors may be required to trust individuals with whom they are not immediately familiar but who function within (and represent) particular institutions – such as those of expert knowledge (eg psychiatry) or the welfare state (eg NHS). These broader institutional experiences and perceptions, described as system-trust by Luhmann (1979, 1988), are referred to as *hyphenated* forms of trust by Williamson (1993: 475–9) in that they reflect the attachment of trust in its looser sense to certain broader social phenomena: the socio-cultural; politics; regulation and professionalisation; corporate culture; and networks. It would seem essential to ensure that our analyses of specific decisions and processes regarding transactions (in relation to their trusting or calculative aspects) are sensitive to the broader system processes that are drawn upon in individuals' decision-making and in which the knowledge applied in decisions is embedded (see Chapter Five).

Socio-cultural trust

Beginning with *context* in its widest form, general socio-cultural tendencies will shape the nature of interpersonal reactions and thus influence trust within particular macro-spheres. Williamson (1993: 476) uses the well-acknowledged contrast between the high levels of trust and taken-for-granted common norms that have been described as a feature of Japanese business transactions and those of southern Italy. These reflect similar descriptions of the differing levels of social capital between certain southern regions in Italy and others further north (Putnam, 2000: 345) and the especially high levels of norm-based social order, mutual visibility and trust in Japan (Sztompka, 1999: 94). Our application and definition of trust (see Chapter One) is far narrower than certain studies that include social capital under a broad umbrella of 'trust'; yet the socio-cultural features of a society by which, for example, rules are adhered to and reciprocal behaviour does not depend upon calculation can be seen to enable broader assumptions about the consistency of human action upon which more specific future expectations (trust) can be built (Sztompka, 1999). In contrast, where basic norms and tenets of social interaction are not experienced as reliable and comprehensible, the result is antithetical to trust: 'vicious circles [where] nearly everyone feels powerless, exploited, and unhappy' (Putnam, 2000: 345).

Not only do *inter*-country differences exist, but Williamson (1993) also denotes features of specific minority ethnic groups (eg Jewish diamond traders in Manhattan) and their own normative interaction codes that facilitate trusting behaviour. However, these shared norms can be viewed as relating to *intra*-minority interactions while divergent *inter*-ethnic norms, and connected limitations to the intelligibility and predictability of interactions, can do much to undermine trust between ethnic communities and therefore the experiences of minority ethnic groups in healthcare settings (Calnan and Rowe, 2008: 22). Appelby (2008) notes the decidedly negative experiences and low levels of trust between certain minority ethnic groups and mental health services in the UK. Such generalised distrust can be understood as developing out of a history of negative interactions with services, but may also be located within more general power dynamics, cultural experiences of inequality and resulting norms of interaction operating across society as a whole (Sztompka, 1999).

These multilayered socio-cultural contexts, operating across national and regional levels, as well as within the more specific contexts experienced by particular minority ethnic groups within certain urban locales, can all be seen as 'fields' (Bourdieu and Wacquant, 1992), which are relevant to the processes by which certain attitudinal and behavioural dispositions are inculcated. The forming of such aspects of habitus has been seen as relevant to people's general tendencies to trust (Misztal, 1996; Scambler and Britten, 2001), or mistrust, and this offers a useful framework for connecting tendencies within the actions of individuals to broader macro-processes that are manifest across society (for an extension of these notions pertaining to trust habitus, see Chapters Three and Five).

Political trust

The significance of inequality between groups also points to the bearing of the political on trust. This begins with Putnam's considerations of the reliability of institutions and the observation of laws/rules, but extends towards the experiences of certain individuals and groups within a state and their corresponding practices of citizenship. Where individuals' relations and perceptions towards the state, and its institutions, affirm a sense of citizenship, inclusion and of being valued, they are encouraged to interact with institutions in a particular, trusting, format that is likely to be conducive to positive outcomes. In stark contrast, Appelby (2008: 402) relates to meeting:

> young Caribbean men who view mental health services as a branch of the criminal justice system, just another place where they can be held in custody. That is a terrible thing to have to admit and an urgent problem to put right.

Here, the broader experiences of inequalities in relation to the 'abstract system' of the state as a whole are extended into specific interactive experiences (Giddens, 1990).

Taylor-Gooby (2008) links these forms of citizen-relationship between local communities and states to the policy frameworks developed by the latter.

Focusing on trends within UK policymaking that reflect developments discussed in preceding sections, he argues that the implicit understanding within these frameworks is dominated by rational actor models that are too narrow to consider the significance of reciprocity – therefore alienating certain already marginalised groups and damaging public trust overall. This leads public institutions, particularly those within the welfare state, to conceive of and thus treat 'clients' within certain procedural formats and based on certain logics of behaviour. As a result, these institutions may function more efficiently, but the narrowly instrumental conception of action – an impoverished awareness of 'the social' that is devoid of norms, values and emotions – renders 'a system that may work better but is trusted less' (Alaszewski and Brown, 2007: 9).

Regulatory and professional trust

The role of appropriate and successful regulation is a further background source of beliefs in levels of competence and fiduciary motives that can facilitate trust in specific situations. This is especially the case with professions, whose very existence, power and relationship with the state and society function through the process of licensing and regulation – both self-regulation and external – as a means of ensuring public trust in professional practice (Salter, 1999). Changes to the 'self-' and external regulatory processes over the past decade have thus been a response to concerns by the public and policymakers about the motives and competency of doctors, as constructed through inquiries and corresponding media and political interest. Meanwhile, survey measures of public trust in the medical profession remain consistently high (MORI, 2004).

A small number of high-profile inquiries in other areas of medicine have driven changes to procedures of self-regulation (eg revalidation), while psychiatry is subjected on a relatively regular basis to the compulsory investigations that take place following a homicide committed by a service user (Warner, 2006). In line with societal demands for the consequences of decisions to be made more calculable/risk-oriented, media reportage in the light of these inquiries has demonstrated an increasing tendency to blame individual professionals, particularly psychiatrists, for failings and fatalities (Hallam, 2002). There is little data as to whether these reports impact on public trust in psychiatry, though they have certainly driven policy reforms (Brown, 2006).

In any case, mental health services in England are prone to depictions and perceptions of underfunding, poor-quality care and failing to protect service users and the public from risks associated with psychosis (Burns and Priebe, 1999). The generally negative portrayal of psychiatry, mental health services and psychiatric medication (Britten, 1998) in the public sphere, in recent media accounts and across a very chequered history, alongside the enduring stigma that taints those who are in contact with services, would also seem to ward against trust (for a fuller discussion of these themes, see Chapter Two). Changes to professional self-regulation and external frameworks such as the CPA would seem impotent, at least in the short term, to rectify this contaminated 'atmosphere'.

Corporate culture and trust

Although dominant caricatures and the history of mental health services offer distinctly problematic foundations for trust, the public sector ethos of NHS mental health services may in contrast be viewed more positively – especially in comparison to other countries. Healthcare arrangements in the United States have been described as placing trust in doctors under threat, from a number of perspectives. Gray (1993) argues that traditional arrangements came to undermine the trust of third-party purchasers of healthcare in clinicians, due to the exceedingly high levels of expenditure and unnecessary use of certain medical procedures. Meanwhile, reforms towards the more efficient/rationed 'managed-care' model have created new tensions in trust, this time from the perspective of patients. Mechanic (1996: 1694) describes the growing awareness and suspicion among patients that doctors may make medical decisions due to the existence of certain rationing incentives rather than the sole fiduciary interest to provide optimum care for the patient: 'Strong financial incentives raise questions about the quality of treatment provided under managed care. But our concern here is less with the actual quality of care than with the trust it engenders.'

In contrast, medical decisions within the NHS, though taken within an implicit rationing system where professionals are aware of limited resources, are arguably less explicitly tainted by direct financial incentives for professionals. While these assumptions may be shifting in the case of GPs, as the financial incentives of the Quality Outcomes Framework attract increased attention within the public sphere, psychiatrists and mental health professionals are more likely to be perceived as driven by a more benevolent public servant ethos. Yet, although there is a lack of apparent financial self-interest on the part of individual mental health professionals, there may potentially be other motives that service users may see professionals as prioritising. An institutionalised preoccupation with risk (Szmukler, 2001) may lead a number of patients to believe that considerations of risk minimisation are likely to be placed ahead of their own concerns – most palpably within the process of sectioning. A more general awareness of the underfunding of mental health services may also suggest an inherent cultural tendency towards pharmaceutical interventions ahead of other forms of therapy.

Networks and trust

Beliefs related to these forms of 'hyphenated trust' – from society at large to the specific institutional culture of mental health services – are ultimately consolidated, or not, in the local social networks of the individuals who come into contact with mental health services. Circles of family, friends, colleagues and other social connections may enforce beliefs that psychiatry is a reliable, incompetent or overstretched profession. Sources of knowledge from within these social networks will vary, from more remote depictions accessed through certain news media – Hallam (2002) notes the attention paid to 'risk and mental health service' topics within the UK broadsheet press in contrast to the tabloid media – to the direct experiences of known relatives or friends with mental health services. In a similar manner to which socio-economic contexts inculcate dispositions and tastes towards certain formats of such media consumption than others, so too may inequality (as related to class, ethnicity, gender and the intersection of these) be useful in considering different perceptions of medical professionals and the NHS – from the deferential to the demanding; from staunch support to scathing cynicism. These different accounts may be woven together to form a tapestry of understanding of the NHS more generally, or mental health services and professionals in particular. Alternatively, a particular network of family and acquaintances may be largely devoid of relevant narratives that influence an individual actor's perceptions – though this is itself a form of disposition inculcated within contexts.

The *direct* social experiences of an actor within a particular local network, particularly in their relationships with direct household/family members, are also likely to be of significance to more general dispositions to trust in that these bear upon an individual's assumptions of the reliability and trustworthiness of others – especially authority figures. Giddens (1990) draws on Erickson's psychological research on early childhood experiences in reaching his definition of 'ontological security', which 'refers to the confidence that most human beings have in the continuity of their self-identity and in the constancy of the surrounding social and material environments of action ... a sense of the reliability of persons and things' (Giddens, 1990: 92). As noted already (and as will be further considered in Chapter Five), recurring social experiences within a person's main social network in later life are also likely to impact on a *habitus* for relating to others in general, one that may be more or less inclined to view certain people – experts, those in authority, those with certain interaction manners – as trustworthy and reliable.

Overview of the book

The preceding section has outlined a number of background contexts to trust and ways in which these may shape the various assumptions and processes that are very central to our study of the concept. Each of these various background features discussed merit significant exploration in their own right. While this is not possible within the confines of this volume, these various contextual influences will continue to surface within the following chapters as we continue to explore the nature of trust amidst heightened vulnerability and uncertainty. The precise format of the book is briefly sketched as follows.

Chapter One will develop a number of the themes raised in this Introduction – especially risk, vulnerability and uncertainty – and develop these in order to come towards a more precise conception of trust in relation to these related factors. Social theories of trust will be drawn upon in achieving this, before we go on to consider the difficulties of researching trust in empirical settings and our own phenomenological approach. We also describe some specific aspects of the empirical research that we draw upon.

Chapter Two will further develop the theoretical/conceptual framework set out in Chapter One, illustrating this in more depth through the qualitative data from our interviews with service users and professionals. Sections will investigate how these respondents – especially service users – reconciled broader assumptions regarding the motivations and competencies of actors (based on institutional context, profession and other ideal-types) with more individualised 'signs' expressed through face-to-face communication. This chapter in particular will consider how trust in individuals is possible despite more problematic institutional contexts.

Chapter Three will tackle some of the tensions alluded to already between conceptions of trust as a more or less 'rational' form of behaviour. A range of arguments that consider trust as more or less calculative, cognitive and emotional, and conscious and less than conscious will be considered in the light of our own findings, and in particular we seek to demonstrate how many of these dualisms that exist within trust research may be overcome within analyses.

Chapter Four tackles another contentious theme that is emerging within the trust literature pertaining to vulnerability, choice and power. Considerations of the extent to which one is able to *choose* a course of action within a specific situation, and the corresponding relevance of trust (or whether the term 'trust' should indeed be applied at all), will be explored.

Chapter Five moves towards considering the more particular organisational and policy setting of our study and especially considers the possibilities and difficulties for trusting relationships to develop within a context dominated by frameworks of risk, calculability and accountability. In particular, we focus on the experiences of professionals and managers in the varying mental health contexts of our study and the manner by which a culture of audit and risk bears upon different relationship dimensions within the organisation.

By way of conclusion, Chapter Six will draw together a number of the key themes emerging within the book and consider these, and the value of trust, as a principle for policymaking, at local and macro-policy levels. Mental health policy has oscillated over many years between facilitating the meeting of need through a more medicalised focus and recurring preoccupations with proceduralism (Jones, 1972) – not least those around risk. We argue that mental health services organised around a concept of trust may be more effective in satisfying both these concerns. The potential for trust to replace risk as a dominant organising concept for mental health policy is thus explored alongside factors that limit such a possibility.

ONE

Investigating trust: some theoretical and methodological underpinnings

Risk, vulnerability and uncertainty

In the Introduction, we outlined a number of features of late-modern societies – uncertainty, complexity and abstractness in particular – which may serve to heighten experiences of anxiety and vulnerability (Wilkinson, 2001) and, moreover, exacerbate challenges to individual considerations of action and decision-making (Beck, 1992). We noted the existence of various processes, connected to the individualisation of society, by which the futures of individual actors are seemingly more contingent on their own decisions than was previously the case (eg pension-planning; see Jones et al, 2010), but where the range of information and expert support is also perceived as more contested, constructed and potentially fallible than before. The existence of decision-related contingencies amidst uncertainty points towards the salience of *risk* within this context – both for individuals as they seek to make decisions in the everyday (Zinn, 2008a) and for policymakers as they attempt to manage institutions in a legitimate, effective and economically viable manner (Kemshall, 2002).

Risk involves the contingency of future outcomes – often referring to negative outcomes, though this is not necessarily so – in relation to the *probability* that a particular outcome will result as well as the *magnitude* of its impact. In this sense, risk is a lens for considering eventualities within an uncertain future and a mode of planning or acting in relation to these. In its narrowest sense, considerations of risk are decidedly calculative ones, involving the refinement of technologies that seek to gauge the probability of certain events (a patient failing to cooperate with psychiatric treatment) and the magnitude of the consequences of this (for the patient and others in the context). However, a number of social scientists, for example Mary Douglas (1992), alongside academics working within mental health services (eg Szmukler, 2003), emphasise various broader considerations that are inherent to how we think about risk. For when we consider future outcomes, as these are attributed to individual decisions (Luhmann, 1993), we are not just thinking mathematically. Rather we are attaching *values* to the perceived outcomes, and this process renders risk a thoroughly political and moral phenomenon as much as a calculative one (Douglas, 1992; Szmukler, 2003).

Yet, while risk is never, and can never be, *purely* calculative, it does nonetheless involve an approach to the future that invokes probabilistic thinking and an assessment of action in the light of this. The invocation of notions of risk therefore assumes that there is a way of drawing on particular, quantified, information from the past and the present as a way of actively managing future outcomes (Alaszewski and Burgess, 2007). Where future outcomes are not able to be causally connected to the present and the past in way that effectively facilitates future planning (Knight, 1921), or where attempts to act in relation to the future avoid calculative approaches (Langlois and Cosgel, 1993), the concept of risk is inappropriate in describing action. Instead, notions of *uncertainty* (and *vulnerability* where potential outcomes are valued as negative) are more appropriate. It is following this type of argument that Zinn (2008a) designs a spectrum between risk-based (more calculative) approaches to the uncertain future and a range of other less-than-calculative bases for acting (see also Williamson, 1993).

Conceptualising trust

What trust is not ...

These distinctions between perceptions of the extent to which uncertain future outcomes are amenable to calculative action or not (risks *versus* uncertainties/unknowns) and associated formats of managing this uncertainty (calculative *versus* less-than-calculative) are highly relevant to the current section where we seek to define the nature of *trust* – as well as distinguishing this concept from what it is not. There is a great deal of ambiguity in the field as regards the plethora of definitions of trust that are used (Barbalet, 2009). When applied at the abstract level, these are impossible to fully reconcile (Pilgrim et al, 2011), yet we hope at the least to be specific about our own terminology and conceptual apparatus, which will facilitate clarity throughout the remainder of the book.

Trust becomes relevant to an actor when there is an awareness of the potential for negative outcomes as a result of acting in relation to, and relying upon, another actor. This awareness of the possibility of 'a bad outcome' is what differentiates trust from confidence – where negative consequences are not even considered (Luhmann, 1979). Yet, in relation to the earlier discussion, we should not say that people trust amidst situations that are 'risky'. If we remain true to the definitions set out in the preceding section, trust is not so much a solution to risk as an alternative. Whereas risk is a highly calculative approach to future uncertainty via categorisable outcomes and probabilistic reasoning (Knight, 1921), trust is an approach that is less-than-calculative – though not entirely absent of calculation (Williamson, 1993) and in many senses decidedly rational (Barbalet, 2009).

There is a burgeoning literature around this tension between the calculative and less-than-calculative components of trusting – where trust is 'both less and more than knowledge' (Simmel, 1990: 179), between rational and non-rational (Zinn, 2008a), between cognitive and affective (Barbalet, 2009), and built on implicit assumptions through the active construction of inferences (Brown, 2009a). Sztompka (1999: 2) notes the general progression away from conceptions of trusters as '"*homo economicus*" ... toward the richer picture including also emotional, traditional, normative, cultural components', yet the rational actor model has continued to be popular, especially in political science and economics. In contrast to some of the more reductivist work within these latter two fields, trust is most usefully, holistically and, therefore, accurately comprehended as encompassing all of the features listed above – rather than a set of '*either/or*' dualisms. For example, Barbalet (2009) and Brown (2009a), drawing on quite different literatures, both denote the role of emotions within trust as a sophisticated format of applying knowledge from prior experiences and, hence, see the 'affective' as one mode of exercising rationality (and knowledge) rather than an alternative to rational modes of decision-making.

So far, we have sought to clarify that trust is thus neither neatly demarcated, nor purely rational-calculative, nor the same as confidence. Two further distinctions we would like to draw are those between trust and the related concepts of familiarity and reliance. As implied earlier, trust as it is considered in this study is a process of acting within a *specific context*, where another person is relied upon and where this reliance could render negative outcomes that would lead to regret (Luhmann, 1979). It is in this Luhmannian sense that trust comes to be seen as quite separate from more general notions of familiarity or social reciprocity: 'Familiarity is an unavoidable fact of life; trust is a solution for specific problems' (Luhmann, 1988: 95). So, while familiarity is important for trust (Adler, 2001), the latter should not be reduced to the former as if trust was simply a matter of knowledge of, or positive dispositions towards, a particular actor (Luhmann, 1988: 94). Such *generalised* views or expectations linked to familiarity or social reciprocity – a form of Williamson's (1993) 'hyphenated trust' – lack an association to a particular set of circumstances but, moreover, mask over the notion of *choice* that is inherent to trust (Luhmann, 1988). Some degree of choice is essential for trust to be relevant. Without a necessary decision and resulting contingency, an actor is merely in a position of reliance or dependence (Meyer and Ward, 2009).

For Luhmann (1979), it is these notions of contingency and complexity – which are bound up with *choice* – that drive us to the very heart of trust. Choice is thus essential for trust but, as some authors have questioned, where a truster is highly dependent on a person or service (especially in healthcare contexts), choice may be rendered unviable and accordingly notions of trust may be irrelevant (Meyer and Ward, 2009). These concerns are central to the content of Chapter Four. For now, it is sufficient to note that dependence does not necessarily preclude choice and therefore trust can still be salient. Indeed, for certain significant authors within the recent literature, notions of dependence (Barbalet, 2009), or of making oneself vulnerable to another (Möllering, 2006), are very much inherent to the trusting process.

Trust as a response to uncertainty amidst vulnerability

Thus far, we have discussed a number of conceptual distinctions around that which trust is not. Before we proceed to clearly define what trust *is*, we seek to paint a more detailed picture of the 'specific problems' to which Luhmann refers – the contexts in which trust becomes relevant. Central to the understanding of trust applied in this study is the relation of the concept to notions of vulnerability and uncertainty (Möllering, 2006). Indeed, if the situations and problems where trust is relevant in our study share one common feature it is this – the concomitant existence of vulnerability and uncertainty and the experienced need of actors (eg service users and professionals) to overcome/manage these conditions.

The complexity of the linkages between these three concepts – trust, uncertainty and vulnerability – is an obstacle to straightforward, neat analyses of trust, but also imperative to effective understandings. As noted in the Introduction, uncertainty is associated with vulnerability (eg uncertainty itself can foster anxiety, which is associated with vulnerability). Trust, meanwhile, is a response to uncertainty about the future – a process that facilitates action in spite of incomplete knowledge. More specifically, though, it is important to reiterate that uncertainty in itself does not require trust. Trust becomes useful when actors concomitantly experience uncertainty *and* vulnerability.

Vulnerability is thus a necessary precondition to contexts where trust is potentially applied (Barbalet, 2009) – but, moreover, the process of trusting involves the actor making him- or herself vulnerable to the actions of the trustee. In this way, vulnerability is both a condition for, and an outcome of, the trust process (again this paradox will be returned to in Chapter Four) as the actor seeks to achieve a particular outcome:

> Trust is understood in terms of a) acceptance of dependency in b) the absence of information about the other's reliability in order to c) create an outcome otherwise unavailable. The first of these is the cost of trust; the second, the situation of uncertainty it faces and may overcome; the third, its purchase. (Barbalet, 2009: 367)

The problem of uncertainty faced by the truster is not singular but multilayered – although these layers are very much interconnected. First, there is the uncertainty as to the potential achievability of the outcome (eg the effective management of psychotic symptoms); and, second, the suitability of the solution to be pursued is also an unknown. The complexity around these first two concerns may be resolved through trust in a particular agent/expert, yet, third, there is uncertainty over the trustworthiness of this actor. Fourth, even if the truster is convinced by the apparent trustworthiness of the trustee, Barbalet (2009: 368) notes one further problem – that of self-trust:

> Most treatments define trust in terms of a confident expectation regarding another's behaviour. We shall see that this covers only half of its mechanism as it leaves out the essential component of a self-referential confidence in the subject's own judgement or appraisal of the other's qualities.

It is helpful to clarify these multiple layers of uncertainty faced by the truster, partly in order to offer a more specific account, but, furthermore, because it illuminates the salience of the specific case under study to more general considerations of trust. Whereas some of these four layers remain hidden or implicit within a number of empirical explorations of trust, interactions between mental health service professionals and service users with diagnoses of psychosis bring all these levels of uncertainty into vivid relief:

1. The chronic, enduring nature of many service users' experiences of serious mental health problems places the achievability of a positive outcome, or even the conception of what a positive outcome might look like, into doubt. Professionals and service users may have quite different considerations as to what 'recovery' might mean. Moreover, short-term successful management in the past may often have been followed by relapse, and thus positive expectations regarding longer-term outcomes may be undermined.
2. The psycho-pharmaceutical approach to service users' symptoms, which is the basis of the vast majority of interventions (for the service user participants in our research and more generally), may often have been experienced as ineffective and/or negative in the past. As a result, expectations regarding the potential for this means of intervention to bring about a successful outcome may be problematic; highly problematic in certain cases.
3. While trust in particular professionals – those providing regular support and those prescribing – may overcome these intervention uncertainties, there are a number of reasons why trust in mental health professionals may be less straightforward than in other areas of healthcare. Brown and colleagues (2009: 453) suggest that there may be particular uncertainties over the interests of these professionals – due to perceptions of their prioritising risk ahead of patient concerns (as potentially experienced by service users who have been sectioned in the past). Moreover, these authors point towards 'the continued status of mental health as the "Cinderella service"' (Joint Committee, 2005) of the NHS, and that this is also likely to compromise beliefs around the capabilities and competencies of agencies to meet their needs (either in the community or as inpatients) (for a further discussion on perceptions of institutions and problems of trust, see Chapter Two).
4. Finally, and particularly relevant within our research context, is the issue of 'self-trust', which Barbalet (2009) underlines as a vital component to the process of trust and one neglected within much of the literature. Across the small corpus that does recognise this feature, we can elucidate two separate, though related, dimensions: one more specific to confidence in one's ability to appraise the likelihood of future outcomes (Barbalet, 2009); the other a more profound 'confidence that most human beings have in the continuity of their self-identity and in the constancy of the surrounding social and material environments of action … a sense of the reliability of persons and things' (Giddens, 1990: 92). Giddens sees this latter ontological security as an important basis for daily

life and trust decisions, specifically referring to paranoid schizophrenia as an example of where this basic confidence is undermined. While we do not want to rush to such an assumption, and see this as an empirical matter for investigation, there may be particularly deep levels of uncertainty experienced by people experiencing severe mental health problems in this regard. There is also literature which suggests that the former aspect of self-trust – that pertaining to confidence in specific interpersonal judgement – may also be problematic for the service users in our study. Trust in one's own cognition, not least in terms of ability to make 'social judgements' (Baas et al, 2008), may be temporarily destabilised among some of those experiencing certain forms of psychosis (Couture et al, 2008).

These multiple and heightened levels of uncertainty, combined with potentially significant levels of vulnerability – for example due to the stigma of mental illness, which contact with psychiatric services reinforces alongside perceptions of treatments and interventions as intrusive and unwelcome – help underline the relevance of our study to illuminating important issues around trust (as we have stated earlier). Moreover, we view this study as an important step towards developing understandings of the nature of trust relations within mental health services, seeking to build upon the small number of studies currently published (for a useful review, see Laugharne and Priebe, 2006). It should be added that not only are service users facing high levels of uncertainty, but also mental health professionals are dealing with significant ambiguities, not least in terms of diagnosis and prescribing (Kirk and Beahrs, 1986; Kutchins, 1992), which are less tangible and precise than in most other domains of healthcare. Hence, the salience of trust reaches beyond simply the experiences of service users and is relevant right across the concerns of professionals and the efficacy of management.

Defining trust: a problem of knowing

In this chapter thus far, we have delineated certain aspects of what trust is not, while also setting out an understanding of the uncertain and vulnerable contexts in which trust becomes relevant. In this section, we now turn our attention to a conceptualisation of trust that will form the basis of the analysis in later chapters. As the uncertainty outlined in the preceding section points towards, trust in many of its senses is ultimately to do with a problem of knowing – of how confident expectations pertaining to a future outcome can be made in spite of incomplete knowledge about the trustees who are depended upon in order for this outcome to be realised (Barbalet, 2009). In developing how this process of 'expectation formation' is achieved, our analysis is arranged around four key components to trust: as an *active construction* of inferences; facilitated through a *relational process*; enabled by the civilising *structuring of social action*; and inherently involving the *bracketing off of uncertainty*.

Trust as an active construction of knowledge

Although the multiple complexities, contingencies and thus uncertainties denoted in an earlier section of this chapter may be unusually elevated in the settings explored in our study, there nonetheless exist manifold contexts encountered by individuals in everyday life where calculation is an inappropriate, insufficient and/ or inefficient approach to complex uncertainties, and, hence, trust is necessary (Zinn, 2008a). The insufficiency of knowledge derived from past experience for coordinating action towards the future helps elucidate the weakness of narrow rational choice models of trust (eg Coleman, 1983; for a critique, see Hardin, 1992[1]) due to the limitations of inductive knowledge (Simmel, 1990) and the corresponding requirement for alternative accounts of knowledge formation.

The conceptualisation of trust as a social process, and, moreover, as a process involving the development of knowledge or beliefs, indicates the potential utility of exploring the concept through a theoretical framework that is grounded within Schutzian phenomenology (Brown, 2009a). Schutz's (1972) prime concern is the social construction of knowledge, and, hence, his understandings of how actors infer knowledge from social contexts and weave these into intricate understandings of other actors within the social world would seem highly relevant to trust. From this phenomenological perspective, therefore, trust is a process of building over, or 'bracketing' away (Sartre, 1962 [1939]), that which is uncertain or unknown through a process of inferential constructs based on that which *is* known. In this sense, trust is neither purely inductive nor deductive; rather, by way of its development as a process and ongoing experience over time, it is more accurately reflected by an abductive model of 'knowledge' development (Danermark et al, 2002).

The conception of trust as a process of constructing knowledge helps draw attention to the *active* role of the truster. Certain empirical analyses of contexts where people trust place significant explanatory emphasis on the qualities of the trustee, yet the truster is certainly highly significant (Barbalet, 2009) and has much agency (Khodyakov, 2007). Barbalet (2009) draws our attention to the self-referential and reflexive activities of trust, while a phenomenological perspective emphasises the contingency of trust on the creative qualities of the truster as she draws upon a multitude of knowledge sources and builds a framework of inferences that bridge the uncertainties faced. Brown and colleagues (2011b: 288), for example, note how patients with the same consultant surgeon drew on quite different aspects of this professional's 'presentation-of-self' in inferring the qualities they saw as appropriate in order for them to develop positive expectations regarding their treatment amidst the experience of cancer.

Trust as a relational process

A number of more recent accounts of trust emphasise a range of ways in which trust is less a 'one-off' decision, although it may involve particular decisive moments of choice, and more an ongoing process (Khodyakov, 2007) within which certain passages of time are apparent (Barbalet, 2009). Two particular temporal frames are significant for the relationship between the truster and the trustee. The first involves the interactions up to and including the particular context where trust becomes relevant (ie a decision is made to make oneself vulnerable to the actor for a future outcome). It is in these interactions that the trustee performs (wittingly or otherwise) a presentation-of-self from which the truster makes a number of interpretations as to the 'latent intentionality' and competency of the truster (Brown et al, 2011b) that are vital for trust.

The second significant temporal frame is described by Barbalet (2009) and pertains to the time between the context where the truster chooses to make himself vulnerable and the moment where the outcome (around which trust was invested) is realised or not. This is the passage where the truster faces multiple vulnerabilities – including both the initial vulnerability that warranted trust in the first place and the added vulnerability due to the potential for being let down by the trustee (see Chapter Four).

Hardin (1992) uses the term 'thick relationships' in reference to the length and depth of relationships that are typically referred to as the basis of trust – although, as he notes, there are a number of sources from which knowledge can be drawn (and trustworthiness inferred) other than these. Broader institutional sources of knowledge will be explored in the next main section (and in more depth in Chapter Two), but there is also a literature around the phenomena of 'swift trust' (Dibben and Lean, 2003), by which family doctors, for example, and other health practitioners may win trust through very short, though highly-skilled, interactions. Hence, although sustained relationships may offer a degree of familiarity that is conducive to trust, effective communication by the professional – both verbal and non-verbal – is able to win trust within decidedly short relational periods (Brown, 2009a).

Trust made possible through structuration

Open, two-way communication is significant to trust in healthcare professionals due to the requirement that the professional demonstrates characteristics of 'competence and care' (Calnan and Sanford, 2004: 96), but also because of the need for the service user to have the opportunity to articulate the outcomes they seek: 'For how can a patient be assured that his/her best interests are central if they have not had adequate opportunity to convey these interests and voice their concerns?' (Brown, 2009a: 393). The response of the professional within these embodied, communicative interactions is significant: where the presentation is interpreted as demonstrating an attentiveness to the service user's concerns, this may be held to demonstrate their embeddedness within normative frameworks of communicative rationality and 'patient-centredness'. In contrast, poor presentation may suggest the professional's distraction or preoccupation with other interests; this may then be interpreted as evidence of the professional's embeddedness in more instrumental frameworks of bureaucratic efficiency and/or risk management (Brown et al, 2011b).

This approach to trust follows Möllering (2005) in considering that it is these normative frameworks that make trust possible. In this sense, Möllering argues that trust is concerned with far more than mere expectations of the actions of the trustee. Indeed, the future attitudes and actions of individuals are never really knowable. Instead, it is the normative frameworks in which the trustee's actions are embedded that facilitate a dimension of control in relation to the expected outcomes, thus offering a semblance of predictability that enables trust. Within late-modern, scientific-bureaucratic healthcare settings, professionals may find themselves embedded within contrasting frameworks – for example, those driven towards bureaucratic-instrumental efficiency and effectiveness on the one hand, and those oriented to patient concerns and holistic care on the other (Brown, 2008b).

Depending on the concerns of the truster, some sort of balance between the instrumental (competent and effective) and communicative (patient-centred and caring) is ultimately necessary. Effective communication on its own is not sufficient for trust in the longer term if quality outcomes are not also forthcoming. Thus, we can understand the manner by which knowledge is inferred from experiences with a particular professional, in the forming of expectations regarding their future actions, as involving two key assumptions: the embeddedness of the caring professional within norms of quality interaction and care-giving; and, moreover, the commitment of the competent professional within norms of high-quality practice and the attainment of outcomes. Within an ongoing series of communicative instances, the professional's actions are inferred as indicating: (a) which normative framework(s) (s)he is embedded within; and (b) the depth of this embeddedness. Within this inferential framework (a) suggests the likely nature of their future actions and (b) points towards the 'predictability' or presumed consistency of their behaviour.

'Bracketing off' uncertainty through emotions

Predictability is used in inverted commas in the preceding subsection as, of course, it remains decidedly tentative. Nonetheless, the norms that orient action, and which exist in heightened form around professional work (Barber, 1983), are active in exerting potent sanctions (of shame and guilt) in incidences where trust is significantly betrayed and, therefore, can be seen as an important part of a 'civilising process' (Brown and Calnan, 2011) that regulates and compels professional action in particular directions. Agency that contradicts these normative structures is still possible but at a high cost.

One of the dimensions of this civilising process that would exact such a cost for breaches of trust, through a form of 'moral obligation' (Brown and Calnan, 2011) is the emotional facet of the trust decision. The emotional components of trust have been recognised across many different approaches (Zinn, 2008a;

Pilgrim et al, 2011), though it is Barbalet (2009: 374) in particular who draws our attention to 'the capacity of emotion to underwrite trust [as a] forced option in which, through the absence of relevant information, action can only occur if there is a commitment to act. Commitment always involves both emotional apprehension and emotional engagement'. Thus, the trustee's awareness of the truster's apprehension, alongside the mutual sharing in an emotional engagement, places a further emotional and moral obligation on the trustee to act in accord with the fulfilment of the truster's expectations.

In spite of this 'civilising process' through the power of norms, values and emotions (the lifeworld), a potential for disappointment persists. One key aspect that differentiates trust from other similar emotions, such as hope, is that whereas hope maintains a distinct awareness of potential negative outcomes, those who trust are able to act with more resolutely positive expectations (Brown and Flores, 2011). Inherent to trust, then, is the process of actively 'putting the world in brackets', which Sartre (1962 [1939]: 25) notes as one of the important functions of the emotions. Connected to this *selective* focus (Brown, 2009a) is a certain 'will to trust' – an impulse enabling the 'leap of faith' (Möllering, 2006) or commitment (Barbalet, 2009) that is necessary for trust. This reaction can be seen as emerging out of the negative experiences of the truster amidst vulnerability and the felt need to manage this situation. This leads the truster to draw on resources of 'emotional choice or selection of strategy in the absence of relevant evidence' (Barbalet, 2009: 374).

Relating trust in people to trust in systems

As developed in the preceding section, a phenomenological understanding of trust focuses our attention on the communication between the truster and the trustee, and the manner by which the communicative signs (verbal and non-verbal) of the latter are inferred by the former and so constructed into beliefs about the competence and motives of the trustee. We have also noted how expectations regarding motives (sometimes referred to as 'interests') are made possible through normative frameworks that structure the actions of the truster. A Schutzian perspective thus emphasises the primacy of *interpretation* and inference for trust, where signs are inferred to say something about the intentionality and ability of the trustee – these are then constructed into trust.

Of course, this interpretive act does not and cannot take place within a vacuum. It is inherently social and based on the prior interactive and socio-biographical experiences of the interpreter (Schutz, 1972) and corresponding cultural assumptions as to what particular signs signify – through which (s)he seeks to enter into the meaning of the other (Mead, 1962). The salience of this meaning context, and the importance of normative frameworks in which the trustee's agency is embedded, highlight the way trust is very much related to the institutions in which trustees are embedded. This issue has been the concern of a number of studies within social-scientific approaches to trust in healthcare that have explored the extent to which trust is related to the institution (eg professionalism) and local organisation of particular professionals (Hall et al, 2001; Calnan and Sanford, 2004; Dibben and Davies, 2004). There is a general agreement that both are relevant, but that interpersonal factors are most important. Yet these assessments have often been accompanied by a lack of theoretical understanding as to *why* the interpersonal is a more potent basis of trust, and how the system and the interpersonal relate to one another (Calnan et al, 2006).

Giddens (1991) provides a very useful starting point for these considerations in his analytical concepts of (direct–interpersonal) 'facework' and its relation to 'abstract systems' as an 'access point' to this wider system. In this sense, the facework undertaken by healthcare professionals is interpreted in light of the service user's understandings of the abstract system, while also becoming part of the service user's experience of the system – therefore influencing future perceptions. What is less clear from Giddens' analysis is the level of influence of different types of knowledge within this social dialectic. If empirical research points towards the primacy of the interpersonal, then this remains in need of appropriate theorising – we require an account for the relative weakness of the system for trust.

It is here that the utility of phenomenology becomes especially clear. Other theoretical frameworks, for example Mead's symbolic interactionism or Goffmanian analyses (see Fugelli, 2001), represent excellent vehicles for considering interpersonal interaction and its relation to interpretation and knowledge construction. Schutz's (1972) work, meanwhile, comprises a nuanced account of how social actors comprehend abstract systems (eg the postal system) as well as a way of relating this to their knowledge gleaned from interpersonal interactions. A framework based on these understandings will be developed in greater in detail in Chapter Two, but for now it is sufficient to sketch an outline.

For Schutz, the way individuals access and acquire knowledge, that of individuals and more abstract notions, requires the exercise of schemes of a person's own experiences as an 'interpretative framework' (Schutz, 1972: 83). However, comprehending abstract knowledge of systems requires vastly more ideal-typical inferences and corresponding assumptions, and is more distant and tentative therefore, than interactions that are able to be directly observed and experienced (Schutz, 1972: 194). In this way, facework carried out by professionals provides a more 'concrete' form of knowledge for service users in that relatively few inferential steps are required to comprehend and access it. In contrast, the notion of a large institution – by way of its complexity and abstractness – is a less tangible, more remote, notion that does not resonate with actors in the way interpersonal interactions do.

Moreover, when we consider that trust ultimately relies on people rather than systems, because it is only people who can ultimately solve problems of complexity and uncertainty (Luhmann, 1979), alongside the affective dimensions of trust discussed earlier, it becomes clear that the interpersonal is a more 'solid' source of knowledge through which trust is constructed (Brown, 2009a). However, we should not neglect the role of institutional/systemic factors – such as perceptions of healthcare system efficiency, general expectations shaped by social capital, broader levels of system-trust in professions (and other aspects of 'hyphenated trust', see Introduction) – as vital for how the interpersonal is construed.

Researching trust: epistemology and methodology

The conceptualisation and theoretical framework outlined earlier raises a number of considerations for how trust is best investigated. Ontologically, trust is far from a neat, discrete or commonly agreed-upon entity (Pilgrim et al, 2011) and thus poses a number of practical challenges to researchers in that it eludes straightforward measurement, observation or description (Brownlie et al, 2008). This nebulous ontology has important consequences for the epistemology, methods and research design on which this study is based.

That the concept is associated with certain affective qualities (Barbalet, 2009), is 'both less and more than knowledge' (Simmel, 1990: 179), and acts in allaying the equally indefinite (Wilkinson, 2001) and subjective notion of anxiety (Kierkegaard, 1957), underlines the necessity of a hermeneutic, meaning-centred approach for developing understandings of trust and its underpinnings in the area of mental health. These ambiguities around construct validity, combined with the paucity of existing research in the area of mental healthcare, underline the case for employing qualitative methods. Hence, the analyses presented in later chapters are of data from semi-structured, in-depth interviews with a range of key stakeholders in mental health services – service users, professionals and managers – as well as a carer and a chaplain to offer further insights.

A further word is also necessary regarding the ontology of mental illness that informs our analysis. In contrast to our research into trust in a number of other areas of healthcare, the diagnosis of psychosis is less straightforwardly legitimated and, indeed, was disputed or doubted by some of our respondents. Professionals affirmed the need for a note of caution – as one psychiatrist and clinical lead noted: "*Psychiatry is all about uncertainty*". This ambiguity, combined with sociological critiques of the constructed nature of the categories and understandings by which diagnoses are made (eg Brown, 1987), presented us with a number of considerations when interpreting and analysing the data. We provide here some brief fragments of data (which will be returned to in the analyses of future chapters) as examples:

> "I've never personally been able to trust anyone as far as I can throw them."

This utterance says something regarding dispositions towards trust in that for some individuals, regardless of interpersonal or institutional contexts, trust is unusually difficult. That this service user had a diagnosis of paranoid schizophrenia,[2] and referred to a number of experiences that had been interpreted by professionals as paranoid delusions, helps develop a more detailed contextual picture. Yet this service user also very much disagreed with his diagnosis and we were faced, therefore, with the ethical and paradigmatic concerns of respecting the voice of this participant. *Prima facie* there would appear to be a clear tension here between the potential clarity that a label of 'paranoia' might offer when considering trust on the one hand, and our professional commitments as ethnographers on the other. However, by taking a sociological 'step back', we began to see how this conflict could be resolved.[3]

If we begin with more socially oriented understandings of mental illness, we can see how disinclinations towards trust may be embedded within negative and/or traumatic experiences. These form highly 'concrete' bases of knowledge from which future expectations towards others are derived. Hence, a disinclination to trust can be seen as a product of social context rather than mere neurological or psychological 'dysfunction'. The relationship between power, marginalised experiences (eg in relation to migration) and psychosis (Pilgrim et al, 2011) add further credence to an assessment that a propensity towards mistrust is a cogent response to oppressive, unpredictable and/or dysfunctional contexts. Even at the level of neurological functioning, recent research points to the links between experience of oppression and changes to dopamine neurotransmission associated with schizophrenia (Murray, 2008). Within this socially constructed approach, we are able to argue that specific labels are less important to our interpretation of data than the experiences of social context that our participants described in interviews.

It is important, however, that these labels are not completed disregarded. Diagnoses were not only useful in understanding the stigmatising effects of psychosis–related labels (especially schizophrenia) and their impact on service users (Link et al, 1989), but were also applied within participant narratives, occasionally in refuting diagnoses, but often as an effective format of sense-making – as tools in understanding their experiences within particular social environments – for example:

> "When I am manic and becoming really high, I walk on the white lines down the middle of the road ... and I watch out for the attack from behind ... and any male becomes a potential enemy. I become obsessively wary."

In this instance, a service user participant expressly utilises his bipolar diagnosis in describing certain types of experience where trust was especially problematic for him during certain phases. Yet, even here, the gendered aspect of the reaction underlines that while psychological considerations may be relevant in this setting, these are fundamentally related to, and develop out of, the social environment and a much broader socio-biographical experience. Thus, the approach of our study in general, and analysis in particular, is predominantly influenced by constructionism – in terms of the social dialectic of Berger and Luckmann (1966). In this framework the subjectivities inherent to social experiences produce an objective social reality which is then internalised by actors (Berger and Luckmann,

1966). This internalising process means that actors are constrained by their social environment, while also contributing to and modifying this same environment by their actions. The dynamics of these processes will be seen more or less implicitly within our discussion of the different trust dimensions within mental health services in Chapter Five.

The analysis discussed earlier involved qualitative data from 23 interviews that took place throughout 2010 with stakeholders across three contrasting mental health services within one local health authority (NHS Mental Health and Partnership Trust) in southern England. These interviews involved eight service users, the managers of each of the three services, 10 professionals including the clinical leads of each service (two consultant psychiatrists and one consultant psychologist), and at least one social worker and one community psychiatric nurse in each service. These data were accompanied by further insights from interviews with one carer and one senior chaplain. The data from this particular study are those focused upon and discussed in the later chapters of this book; however, the broader analysis and theorisation presented here is also informed by the research of a very insightful colleague (Scrivener, 2010) and the excellent study of a postgraduate student (Maidment et al, 2011).

While the size of our research was comparatively modest, the features of these healthcare contexts that we were exploring – pertaining to experiences of uncertainty and vulnerability and outcomes related to risk and trust – relate to much broader phenomena that are relevant across mental health service contexts and, indeed, late-modernity. Of course, there are a number of limitations to the sample within our study that limit what we can say empirically about mental health service provision more generally, yet we argue that the embeddedness of the micro-social processes that we investigate within a larger-scale social picture (Inglis, 2010) enables our modest case study to say something more broadly relevant:

> The task is to combine an understanding of the emotions, choices and interactions of individuals with an understanding of the social and cultural organizations and structures through which they have been constituted and, consequently, realize themselves as individuals.... Given the principle that elements of the whole can always be found in the part, when these clues are carefully analysed, they can provide an insight into the wider social structure. (Inglis, 2010: 514–15)

In this manner, ethnographic fragments can provide vital insights into more general social processes, thus proving useful starting points of theorisation; although, of course, further refinement and cross-case analysis is necessary to build and refine any theorisation.

Some central analytical foci

A more detailed account of the design, analysis and ethics of the main study, along with brief overviews of these two other studies, is provided in Appendix 1. We finish this chapter by discussing the main considerations of the research that forms the empirical backbone of many of the later discussions in the book.

The underlying purpose of our research was to explore the nature of trust in this context of heightened vulnerability and uncertainty. Moreover, we investigated how trust, distrust (lack of trust) or positive mistrust influenced outcomes – primarily for service users, but also for professionals and managers. Our research in other areas (Calnan and Rowe, 2008; Brown et al, 2011b) had indicated that trust relations across one dimension – for example, between managers and professionals – had ramifications for other dimensions – such as inter-professional trust and professional–service user trust. Our analysis was informed by these understandings, alongside a number of other key themes in the literature. While all of these 'sensitising concepts' (Blumer, 1969) are not exhaustively listed here (any pretence at such a comprehensive list would be misleading as there are surely concepts we were unwittingly sensitised through), five key themes are briefly sketched as follows.

Risk and control, as noted already in the Introduction, are significant themes both in the trust literature, but also within recent clinical and organisational approaches to mental healthcare. Risk, as a control-oriented calculative approach to uncertainty, can be seen as contrasting sharply with trusting approaches – the latter adheres to a person-centred approach, while the former 'trusts' in technologies of control. Moves towards bureaucratic and calculative control can also be seen as antithetical to trust (Gellner, 1988) in that these technocratic approaches are rooted in a lack of trust in individuals (Brown and Calnan, 2010) – for example, service users and professionals – and because the practice of the technocratic may impinge upon the reproductions of the norms on which trust is based (Brown, 2008b).

The constructing of ***knowledge frameworks*** (explicit and assumed), which have been seen in this chapter as being fundamental for trust, were also a central focus of the data analysis. The various types of attributes (personal and institutional) that were important for trust or mistrust were closely scrutinised, as were the ways in which beliefs about these attributes were inferred from existing knowledge and experiences of particular professionals and services. Informed by the theoretical framework presented in this chapter, knowledge was conceptualised in a broad range of formats that ranged from institution-oriented to interpersonal, related to various expectations regarding competencies and motivations, and was applied through more cognitive and/or emotional schemes.

The manner by which knowledge is able to be inferred and applied in contexts where trust may be necessary is significantly influenced by the degree of *familiarity* with which the truster perceives the setting and personnel (Luhmann, 1979). This bears importantly on the range and extent of knowledge available to the actor

(Brown, 2009a) as well as the 'internal dimensions' of trust experienced by the truster in terms of ontological security and trust in their own ability to discern the trustworthiness of others (Pilgrim et al, 2011: 44). These theoretical issues led us to explore factors pertaining to consistency of care and length of relationship and the extent to which these were influential (or not) for trust.

This feature of familiarity is just one mode in which *time* is influential for trust. Time is a fundamental consideration of analysis in that the process of trust inherently involves the linking of knowledge derived from experiences within the past to considerations and expectations regarding the future. Moreover, time had also been a vital factor in our previous analyses of trust through the way that the devoting of time by busy professionals was inferred as demonstrating their benevolence and care (eg Brown et al, 2011b). This theme was not pursued directly through questioning, yet a number of service users and other stakeholders raised the notion of time independently, and, hence, it became another key locus of analysis.

Finally, *space* has not been explored in any significant depth in the trust literature; however, one interesting study (Parr and Davidson, 2008) raises the issue when researching trust amidst online communities. Notions of proximity are important to understandings of vulnerability, familiarity and effective communication. Meanwhile, space is also relevant when analysing the association of certain environments with positive or negative outcomes – hence, the location of interactions with regard to power, conviviality, familiarity and accessibility, as well as the relating of certain spaces to positive or negative emotions, are all potentially relevant when exploring how trust is facilitated or impeded.

Notes

[1] Hardin's position of trust as 'encapsulated interest' is itself criticised by, among others, Pilgrim and colleagues (2011) for being too narrow a consideration of trust. It is argued that this narrow conceptualisation fails to do justice to trust in its broad contextual and relational richness.

[2] We recognise here that the term 'paranoid' in this diagnosis refers more to the presence of positive psychotic symptoms in general than anything specifically to do with paranoid beliefs or delusions.

[3] We are grateful for feedback received on a paper presented at the 2010 British Sociological Association annual Medical Sociology Conference, Durham University. Conversations with David Pilgrim and Ivy Bourgeault, as well as a clinician, Richard Brown, were especially helpful in thinking through some of these concerns.

TWO

Constructing knowledge through social interactions: the role of interpersonal trust in negotiating negative institutional conceptions

This chapter will develop a theoretical framework for understanding how trust in the context of psychosis services is possible – in spite of the emphasis upon more negative characteristics of mental heath institutions within a range of narratives in public sphere discussions and, moreover, within the experiences of many service users. As touched upon in Chapter One, there are a range of potentially significant obstacles to trust in the context of psychosis services and it has been argued that trust, though necessary, would appear *prima facie* unlikely (Brown et al, 2009: 453). First of all, we survey a range of sources of knowledge about services – and the *institution*[1] of psychiatry – which may be drawn upon by service users in contexts of vulnerability and uncertainty, and which accordingly shape the likelihood of processes of trust, distrust or mistrust. The central section of the chapter will then, drawing on Schutzian phenomenology and a typology of knowledge formats outlined by Habermas (1971), develop a framework for understanding the varying significance of different types of knowledge for trust. This will be useful in understanding why, despite negative institutional perceptions and problematic personal experiences, a number of participants in our study described their experiences of relationships within services in terms of high levels of trust.

Three sources of negative institutional conceptions

Psychiatry: history and media portrayals

In a number of senses, 'psychiatry' is an overly narrow heading for this subsection as, of course, modern mental health services include social workers, community psychiatric nurses (CPNs) and psychologists (alongside various other professions allied to medicine such as occupational therapy) and are thus profoundly multidisciplinary. And yet, although doctors make up only a small proportion of the professionals with whom service users are in contact, their influence, profile and history, nonetheless, looms large within general perceptions of the nature of care for people experiencing severe mental health problems, as well as within a number of connotations associated with labels such as schizophrenia and bipolar. The power of the psychiatrist in diagnosing and sectioning[2] and their central role in prescribing decisions renders their presence and reputation as fundamental for how mental health services are viewed within the public sphere.

General public conceptions of mental health services and their portrayal in the public sphere are decidedly, albeit not solely, psychiatry-oriented. The troubled history of the asylum, though notably impacted upon by other professions – not least the legal profession (Jones, 1993) – is in many senses associated with psychiatrists, as are the range of inhumane treatments developed in the name of medicine, an array of contested diagnoses and the considerable side effects of anti-psychotics (Cooper, 1967; Rogers and Pilgrim, 1991; Crossley, 1998). Crossley (1998: 878) notes that 'psychiatry has been an object of criticism and contestation throughout its history' and one recent variant of such criticism has been the portrayal of the flawed decision-making of psychiatrists within official inquiries and media reporting of homicides committed by people in contact with mental health services (Eastman, 1996; Hallam, 2002).

The blaming of experts for failings, a product of the risk-characterised environment (Luhmann, 1993) in which mental health services are currently located, is part of a broader portrayal of mental health services that is highly skewed towards emphasising dysfunction (Burns and Priebe, 1999) and would seem to be especially unfavourable in the UK (Huang and Priebe, 2003). These two negative narratives – of the shambolic institution or system on the one hand (Burns and Priebe, 1999), and of the flawed and incompetent professionals who work within this system on the other – mean that the initial views of those referred to this abstract system are unlikely to reflect the 'ongoing positive feedback' that Luhmann (1979: 50) describes as the basis of 'system trust'. Such negative news media portrayals combine with fictional media representations to depict a decidedly untrustworthy impression of mental health services for future (and current) users. The following quotation is a more severe example of the initial views described by users before their contact with services, but underlines the significant problems of trust in this area of healthcare compared with many others[3] (see also Helene Hem et al, 2008):

> "I was absolutely terrified. The first time I had an appointment to see a psychiatrist I ran away and I went running off and my mum had to chase after me because I was scared at what they would do to me. I had visions of, like, men in white coats coming in and holding me down and forcing medication through my mouth – and they were going to lock me up." (*Service user 7*)

Stigmatising labels and contamination

If fictional and news media portrayals represent significant barriers to the access and trust of mental health services, the potential experience of stigma is another example of an immediate obstacle that is influential before any contact with services has been made. Clearly visible within our interview data was a wariness of services due to concerns regarding the stigma that would result from being referred to mental health services in the first place, especially when receiving prescribed medication. Hence, for some participants,[4] regardless of the quality of their care, there was an inherent negative outcome attached to being in contact with mental health services. While this consciousness of stigma might not provide any knowledge about the attributes of the service and quality of care that would normally relate to trust, fear of labels and the connotations that surround them nonetheless can precipitate an emotional reaction that would bear negatively upon expectations and experiences:

> "I was quite frightened. I was quite frightened by the fact that it was early intervention for *psychosis* [participant's emphasis]. I mean the name itself is a bit....Yes, very reluctant." (*Service user 6*)

Fears related to the future impact of being labelled bipolar, or particularly schizophrenic,[5] were thus detrimental to initial considerations and experiences of mental health services. Labels of riskiness and *otherness*, relating in many senses to stigmatisation, are associated by Douglas (1992) with notions of contamination. In this sense, an outcome of 'dirtied' or spoiled identity (Goffman, 1963), which will live with the individual (by group attribution) regardless of a specific diagnosis or treatment, is intrinsically linked to considerations of service engagement:

> "And that [referral] has some problems attached to it as well because it would be ... obviously any contact with mental health services has a certain degree of stigma attached to it so if we were to see somebody and we were to accept somebody for care coordination who then later doesn't go on to develop psychosis then there's still the stigma of: 'Well, you were cared for by mental health services', and what does that mean and ... about your person as you're developing [as a young adult]." (*Consultant psychologist*)

Previous experiences of mental health services

The first two subsections have referred to negative perceptions of mental health services that are products of potent socio-cultural categories and similarly powerful media-led social constructions within the public sphere that exist *a priori* to interaction with services. Of course, another vital source of information that shaped our participants' perceptions and expectations of services was their own direct experiences. The eight service users we interviewed had been in contact with services for a mean duration of 15.9 years (standard deviation = 12.4) and, hence, many of them had a vast range of experiences, often across an array of different services. In contrast to our research into trust in several other domains of healthcare (where references to problematic or dysfunctional situations were relevant for only a small minority), *all* of the service user participants referred to decidedly negative experiences, which led to severe misgivings regarding the competence and/or motives of professionals working for mental health services in some cases – especially in relation to inpatient settings:

> "There was one particular girl kept badgering me and I went until I couldn't stand no more of this,'I must go to the police' [I was thinking] so I picked up the telephone and asked for the police. I just got through and she came … she was watching me and she grabbed the phone out of my hand, put it down and she grabbed hold of my hair and she said 'You're not gonna tell anybody, just behave yourself'." (*Service user 5*)

> "It's almost like you take, I don't know, 25 sessions and you get somewhere and you could have done the same thing in three." (*Service user 6*)

These previous experiences of services, either as an inpatient (former example) or community-based service user (latter), several years before (former) or within recent months (latter), were significant for participants in shaping their expectations about their future well-being in relation to their contact with mental health services and the likelihood of positive outcomes.

In many cases, these more problematic experiences, from the frightening to the frustrating, were significant in understanding service users underlying assumptions – especially in novel situations where they encountered either a new professional or a new service. Giddens (1990) points to the relevance of general assumptions regarding abstract systems that are extended into specific situations of vulnerability and uncertainty, and thus trust becomes relevant. In contrast to many people encountering other forms of healthcare, the initial assumptions of our service users were either negative in nature or, at the least, highly aware of the potential for unsatisfactory outcomes or loss of control (Dew et al, 2007).

Following Luhmann (1979), and based on distinctions clarified in Chapter One which highlight that trust pertains to specific situations, we should not say that these more general expectations rooted in concrete past experiences indicate a lack of trust. Rather they are most accurately described as a heightened awareness of the potential for negative outcomes from systems that make trust at once both more necessary, but also less likely:

> "Well, I think there are lots of factors [relating to whether service users trust]. Their history with the services, not only mental health services, any services does count. So if they have a good experience, if they have … if they trust the services that will … that gives us … like we are starting on the right foot then." (*Consultant psychiatrist*)

Hence, positive perceptions and 'trust' in the system are significant for understanding the development of trust relations. Yet, as the next section goes on to explore, these institutional views are neither sufficient nor necessary in understanding the development of trust within specific contexts or ongoing relationships (Helene Hem et al, 2008).

Different formats and concreteness of knowledge

As referred to earlier, it is well theorised and empirically established that understanding service user (or patient) trust in healthcare contexts is far from a question of 'the system *or* the doctor', but is, instead, a case of an interrelation between the two (Luhmann, 1979; Giddens, 1990, 1994; Hall et al, 2001; Calnan and Sandford, 2004; Dibben and Davies, 2004; Gilson et al, 2005) – *a dialectic*. Giddens' (1994) conceptualisation of abstract systems and the facework that takes place at the 'access points' to these systems was sketched in Chapter One. It was noted there that although this represents an effective conceptualisation of the interaction between perceptions of systems and encounters within such institutions, a well-developed and systematic theorisation of the primacy of facework and direct experiences (rather than perceptions of the institution) for trust – as has been established empirically through quantitative and qualitative research (eg Calnan and Sandford, 2004; Brown, 2009a; Siegrist, 2011) – is currently lacking.

Anchored in Schutzian phenomenology, the previous chapter also briefly outlined a mode of theorising the greater influence of the interactive for trust – by which the forms of knowledge that are derived from face-to-face communication are more 'concrete' (less reliant on complex inferential frameworks) than the remote, abstract notions pertaining to the system (Brown, 2009a). In order to develop this framework further, it is useful to refer to three different formats of experiential knowledge that may be drawn upon within the construction of trust: mediated, direct-public and interactive-private.

Mediated experiences: 'public' and abstract

Outcome indicator measures that are used widely by healthcare policymakers represent the epitome of 'publicly available' knowledge tools (Habermas 1971: 50) – as opposed to the barely communicable 'private' aspects of experiences. Habermas distinguishes between these forms of account in terms of their generalisability and, therefore, their straightforward accessibility to a large audience of people. The numeric and clearly defined basis on which outcome measures (eg surgical mortality statistics or waiting lists) are developed ensures their potential dissemination to a wide audience and, consequently, their utility in making validity claims about the effectiveness of an organisation (local or national). Yet, although such data are very much generalisable, they are also highly abstract – numbers or graphs on a page with little palpable *experience* apparent within them. Hence, public experiences 'can be expressed in a formalized language, which can be made universally valid by means of general definitions. In contrast, the language of literature must verbalize what is unrepeatable' (Habermas, 1971: 50).

Representations of the NHS in the mass media, while frequently referring to government statistics and other data sources, also tend to use personal stories in order to make their accounts of the institution more *immediate*. The use of emotive language and particular typifications of individual cases (Entwistle et al, 1996) are thus 'capable of "making present" a variety of objects that are spatially, temporally and socially absent from the "here and now"' (Berger and Luckmann, 1966: 174). This selective framing may, therefore, seem more 'real' than a disembodied 'healthcare by numbers' but, nonetheless, occurs at a removed distance from the reader/actor. It, therefore, represents a relatively weak source of experience for the receiver – viewed as it is from a certain distance of abstraction (Brown, 2009a).

Less removed still are those second-hand experiences recounted within the social networks of an individual actor. Whereas a degree of reflexivity would seem to exist towards the selective negativity-bias of mass media reports (Seale, 2003; Pilgrim et al, 2011: 171), the emergence of positive or negative accounts of healthcare via family, friends, work colleagues or other acquaintances is not only less obviously framed, but, moreover, these narratives may also often refer to the same local NHS organisation as that accessed by the person receiving the information. The proximity – geographically or emotionally (if the subject of the story is well known to the receiver) – therefore heightens the profoundness of the experience (even though 'second-hand') in contrast to more remote media representations and enables a form of 'trust' by networks (Lee-Treweek, 2002; Piippo and Aaltonen, 2008).

Direct 'public' experiences: fewer inferences, more concrete

The remoteness of these 'mediated-public' experiences renders their 'reality' or resonance relatively weak when compared with contexts that are directly encountered.[6] A Schutzian perspective (Schutz, 1972) holds that what can be directly observed by patients or service users is, therefore, often more compelling to them than second-hand accounts. Regardless of what may be read or measured about hospital cleanliness, for example, first-hand observations are a more tangible form of experiential evidence for an individual – which is able to override the more tentative knowledge gained from mediated sources (Brown, 2009a); although, of course, it may often be the case that mediated sources raise the spectre of doubt regarding cleanliness or other such issues (eg waiting lists) in the minds of patients in the first instance.

So, while the mediated knowledge that is formed prior to direct experiences will inform initial 'interests' and affect 'modifications of attention' (Schutz, 1972: 196), direct experiences generate more concrete forms of knowledge, in comparison to mediated depictions and related nebulous notions of the system. Meanwhile, these direct observations may well become reference points in the future for generalising about the institution (Giddens, 1994). For if, as suggested already, more abstract concepts (such as 'the NHS') are only comprehensible via direct experiences (Schutz, 1972), then ongoing periods of treatment or visits to NHS institutions (access points) will lay the basis of new, or reinforced, understandings of the abstract system (Giddens, 1990). Acknowledgements of the importance of these direct experiences are visible in the examples noted in policy documents such as *The NHS Plan* (Department of Health, 2000) and include: waiting times, food quality, improved facilities and enhanced referral systems.

Interactive private experiences: the most 'concrete' bases of knowledge

To return to Habermas's (1971) earlier cited distinction between public and private experiences,[7] it is vital to clarify that these are not drawn from separate occasions or instances. Rather, all 'events' can be understood and represented in their private or public senses – although interpersonal interactions (in terms of the facework they comprise) are much richer in the private aspects of experience. For example, an effective provision of palliative care might be represented publicly as a death statistic, or one that involved minimal stated levels of experienced pain. In contrast, the empathy visible within the body language of the nursing staff or the appropriateness of time the family were given on their own with the body (following death) would be labelled as private experiences (Habermas, 1971) – the '*you had to be there*' aspects.

These latter aspects of a patient's healthcare are the least generalisable and measurable – and, hence, the most likely to be overlooked by the audit and outcomes data referred to earlier (Brown, 2008b). Yet these private guises of experience are also the most profound and concrete for trust. For it is only within the often subtle content of service user–professional interactions that the competency and care necessary for trust becomes apparent and verifiable in a significant manner. Within these communicative instances, the agendas of professionals and service users are able to be clarified and synthesised – as is necessary for trust (Brown, 2008b) – but, more importantly, the actions, gestures and more general comportment of the professional are able to corroborate and in this way validate assumptions regarding the capability and willingness of the professional to fulfil this agenda (Brown et al, 2011b).

Hence, it is in these least generalisable, but most social, aspects of experiences that trust is most concretely grounded (Brown, 2009a). These private facets of experiences not only allow the truster to witness – rather than tentatively infer from a distance – the likely quality and effectiveness of healthcare (as with first-hand 'public' experiences), but also to explore and verify the competence and care of the professionals at the access points of the system. Although attitudinal positions related to trust can be said to be affected by all three experiential levels of abstractness (as discussed in the preceding paragraphs), it is this latter, profoundly relational, layer that bears most decisively upon trust.[8] The 'I think' (private aspects) are far more 'real' for service users than the generalised 'they say' notions of mediated accounts (Cornwell, 1985).

Challenges to the framework: exploring the 'trialectic'

Each of these three formats of knowing identified in the preceding subsections are influential on service user trust (and were visible within our data); however, the model developed earlier emphasises that intersubjective, interactive-private formats of experience are more present and tangible – a richer source of information about the 'latent intentionality' (Merleau-Ponty, 1968: 213) of the trustee-actors. Moreover, the private aspects of experiences possess an emotional resonance that is significantly influential for trust (Brown et al, 2011b) – yet is less substantial in the former two formats.

The framework is a useful way of conceptualising the potency of direct experiences over the weaker system-related knowledge as reported in a number of studies, yet there is other research which introduces empirical findings that would appear to run contrary to this conceptualisation. For example, Solbjør and colleagues' (2010) exploration of trust among women with interval breast cancer (cancer diagnosed following a recent negative – ie all clear – result from mammography screening) noted the surprising steadfastness of trust in spite of the system failures that would appear to warrant its demise. A number (though not all) of these women reported a continuing trust in the institution and professionals providing their treatment, in spite of the direct experiences that might have undermined their esteem of the competency and capacity of healthcare experts to deliver positive outcomes. Apparent within these women's accounts were more generalised notions of the effectiveness of the system and an explanatory framework that held that their cases were unusual or exceptions to the rule.

Such findings represent a challenge to straightforward notions that direct experiences are decisive for trust, but can nevertheless be incorporated within the framework – serving to underline the agency in knowledge construction pertaining to trust as well as the interaction between the three knowledge formats. We referred earlier to Giddens' (1994) analysis of the interaction between facework and systems as what can be referred to as a dialectical process. If we replace this two-way interaction with a framework involving our three formats of knowledge, then we have a trialectical process – and more specifically an asymmetrical trialectic (Brown, 2009a: 397) as represented in Figure 2.1.

That the profoundly negative direct-public experiences – such as a false negative diagnosis (Solbjør et al, 2010) or the development of infection due to basic nursing errors (Brown, 2009a: 397–8) – do not necessarily dissolve trust is due to the way that knowledge is selectively derived from these experiences within a particular interpretive framework. Inferences about the competence and motives of professionals associated with such dysfunctions are not made within a vacuum but, instead, within the context of, and in relation to, other experiences and knowledge formats. Where existing knowledge through mediated formats is positively orienting, and where private-direct interactions at access points are also high-quality, then the negative experience of misdiagnosis is more likely to be interpreted as an aberration. Similarly, Brown (2009a: 397–8) describes a cancer patient, who had become infected following nursing errors, who was similarly able to explain this problem away within a framework that insulated her esteem of the surgical team – who were categorised as most significant in overcoming her cancer and seen as separate to this dysfunction.

Figure 2.1: Asymmetrical trialetic of knowledge formats within trust formation

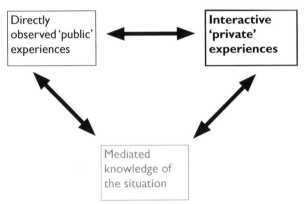

Prevalent within both these examples, therefore, is the colouring of one form of experience (direct-public experiences) by the other two, but where the quality of interactive-private experiences is the most potent – both in building trust and in influencing the inferences made through other formats. These examples also highlight that this process of inference from experiences is a highly active, even deliberative, one (Brown, 2009a) – where continuing trust results from actively 'putting the world in brackets' (Sartre, 1962 [1939]: 25) rather than simply being 'a passive consequence of external attributes' (Brown, 2009a: 402).

Trusting in mental health professionals: distinguishing the individual from the system

The trialectical processes between different formats of experiential knowledge as outlined in the preceding section, combined with the active process of 'bracketing away' aspects of experiences, were clearly apparent within the accounts of the service users and, indeed, professionals in our study. Box 2.1 outlines the experiences and resulting perspectives of one service user who, despite generally negative perceptions of mental health services and highly negative outcomes experienced directly, describes current levels of trust in his care coordinator as particularly high. Corresponding positive expectations in his care are made possible through the development of a highly positive collaborative friendship (Green et al, 2008) – rooted in this professional's exceedingly high-quality interpersonal skills and accompanying demonstration of professional competence. As touched upon in Chapter Three, perceptions of competence and care are often far from two discreet entities,[9] but, instead, are typically bound up with one another in one broader notion of professional 'virtue' (see Pilgrim et ai, 2011).

Within this same account, it is thus apparent that straightforward communicative effectiveness is necessary but not sufficient for the long-term development of trust within this chronic care situation. Outcomes must also be forthcoming in terms of more instrumental or direct-public experiences – such as a reduction in negative symptoms/experiences via helpful medication management. Moreover, the effectiveness of these outcomes is critically dependent upon the work of the care coordinator in developing understandings of the specific expressed needs of the service user. Accordingly, the communicative/private aspects of an experience with a professional may, over time, undergird and enable the achievement of positive experiences in the instrumental/public sense. As these two elements of direct experience interact in a positive manner, so are the previous negative experiences gradually able to be bracketed away. That these negative experiences were direct (rather than mere remote, mediated knowledge about the system) entails that this is neither a quick nor straightforward process. Nevertheless, over time, the concreteness of the facework experiences, and related instrumental outcomes, enables negative past experiences to be bracketed away to a sufficient degree that trust is then able to be developed.

Box 2.1: Trusting in spite of negative experiences

Robert (pseudonym) first came into contact with mental health services almost 25 years ago and has had ongoing contact since then, with six experiences of being sectioned across that time. Over this period, he has become something of an 'expert patient', with significant understandings of his medication and techniques for managing this in order to control his bipolar condition.

He recounted a number of negative experiences as an inpatient. These relate to experiences of care itself – for example:

"I get treated completely different. The staff.... The male staff are frightened of me when I'm in hospital, you can see it. It's partly due to the [ethnicity] stereotypes but it's also because I am high and I am irritated and I am just a pain in the arse."

Moreover, he has been frustrated with not being trusted to manage his own medication in the past, which resulted in unnecessary hospital admissions:

"If somebody's in front of you saying they want to take lithium, lots of it, depacote, lots of it, any benzodiazopene that you've got, lots of it, and halaperadol as much as you can give me – well just read the fucking books. Is that not what you're meant to do people? Five months in there because the tosser, the third guy got me in there in the first place where I could have been here at fucking home."

More recent experiences had also been problematic and frustrating as a result of incompetent and ineffective care coordinators:

"So I've had one man that wasn't there, that was his crime, one woman who wasn't trained and then the third one, the guy who was a nice guy, a bit of a soft gentle guy tried to help and stuff, but [he] wasn't there – and was in well above his level of competence for working in the community with an individual caseload. In as much as he did not know how to prioritise his workload and deal appropriately with emergencies as they cropped up."

Yet, in spite of this long line of inpatient and community care dysfunctions, the most recent care coordinator had proved incredibly effective in terms of both interactive relationship-building (Green et al, 2008) as well as productive outcomes when it came to helping with illness management:

"I can phone her up and tell her how I'm feeling and what's going on and I can say I want to take halaperadol because I'm ... and she'll say don't be daft. She says I'm like that all the time. And she can sort of, just touch base with her and we can just sort of mark where I am. Because she's ... she's a very, very, very busy woman and she's ... she's not going to come in here and fall asleep, you know.... She's alive! That's what I need, see."

In contrast, Box 2.2 refers to the experiences of the one service user we interviewed who referred to an almost utter lack of trust in the professionals with whom he interacted and an overwhelmingly negative view of mental health services overall. For him, a number of negative experiences in the past – not least relating to problematic experiences with police[10] around the time he was first sectioned – had not been superseded by more positive recent experiences. Indeed, his ongoing contact with the assertive outreach team was experienced as compromising his liberty, and he thus continued to experience the facework of the professionals as problematic and seemingly this was partly driven by the assertive context in which these interactions took place:

"Yeah. I mean they will walk in, in any case. They're always in twos at least ... and it's fairly typical that, you know, they will need two or three nurses just to pick on one feeble patient." (*Service user 1*)

In this way, the service context of interactions was an impediment to the type of one-to-one communicative action that might have more adequately built trust. The service user's broader view of the mental health system was also mired by a number of particularly negative experiences with psychiatrists, one in particular, which tainted his view of the service more generally. In this situation, the powerful position of the psychiatrist at the 'access point' would seem to render interactions especially potent in damaging views of the system overall: "The psychiatrist, the man at the top, was corrupt and so the whole kind [of] pyramid was corrupt".

Ongoing problematic interactions with other psychiatrists, who failed to differentiate themselves from the first (in terms of the diagnosis they gave), rendered them all 'contaminated' by the highly deficient and insensitive facework within early encounters:

> "I had this psychiatrist who was so wrong.... I don't believe that they ever listened to a single word I said or, you know, if I said to [this psychiatrist] 'Oh, there's a conspiracy', which it is, and he would just laugh.

> I've just seen too many psychiatrists who all sat there and it seems the doctors just want to broadly agree [with each other]."

Hence, for this service user the power of facework and especially the private experiences of being laughed at and associated feelings of being 'stigmatised and ridiculed', alongside a negative direct-public experience of a diagnosis viewed as incorrect, led to a lack of trust and negative view of professionals in general: "none of them were on my side and I'm not gonna trust any of them".

The lack of any professionals who, perhaps due to the context of assertive outreach work, were able to redress these dysfunctional experiences rendered the service user in a position of continuing distrust. Although he did describe one encounter with a psychiatrist which was much more positive (see Box 2.2), this was seen as the *exception* rather than the norm.[11] This interaction reflected the empathy and pragmatism that Schout and colleagues (2010) note as essential in gaining the trust of those least likely to seek care. Yet, in spite of this one positive episode, the ongoing negative experiences of this service user were too often repeated and concrete for them to be bracketed away.

Box 2.2: Mutuality of accounts amidst a relative absence of trust

David first came into contact with mental health services 10 years ago. This was through a referral following his having been in police custody. This path into contact with mental health services is seemingly problematic as his negative experiences with the police (although he was never found guilty), and their impact on his freedom, are reflected also in his views of the assertive outreach team that he sees as interfering far too much in his day-to-day life:

> "I missed the rent on this place for one month a while ago and the landlord phoned up [the local mental health services] and, you know, said well ... 'Oh, what's going on?'. And of course, you know, mental health services have never been a debt collection agency for any third party, you know, so it's just one example of how people don't realise their remits, as we head towards this nanny state ... you know."

In spite of occasional talk about the possibility of psychotherapy or other interventions, the only intervention open to David has been anti-psychotic drugs. These were initially problematic when prescribed to him as an inpatient:

"And of course I had terrible difficulty sleeping in there, you know, that, you know, under an anxiety state and then anti-psychotic pills….They actually affected my sleep until I was, you know, sleeping one hour a night or something silly and then, you know, you could get the nurse coming in saying why is your light on at night, and things like that."

David referred to a generally negative view of services, and psychiatrists in particular. While he spoke about the staff from the assertive outreach team as being 'nice enough', he talked more generally about his limited trust:

"I've never personally been able to trust anyone as far as I can throw them. You know, and the first things they started writing about me was oh, you know, 'He was very guarded today' and all this sort of thing and of course, you know, none of them were on my side and [so] I'm not gonna trust any of them."

Yet, in spite of these negative perceptions, a lack of trust and resistance to his schizophrenia diagnosis, he continued to take his medication:

"Fortunately, you know, we agree to disagree because I take the psychotic pill to cure anxiety state and they want me to take it for schizophrenia. Fortunately, you know, the end result is the same, we both agree to take the pill for different reasons."

This points towards what O'Neill (1995) describes as a 'mutuality of accounts' – where both 'expert' and 'layperson' adopt a pragmatic position in order to enable conflicting paradigms to overlap sufficiently to enable cooperation. This may be one mechanism whereby cooperative relations are able to develop effectively, even within low-trust contexts.

This one participant aside, all the other service users we interviewed described some degree of trust in the professionals with whom they were currently dealing, with some reporting very high trust indeed. However, in contrast to our research in other contexts, *all* participants referred to times in the past where trust had been problematic (for some, decidedly so). This leads us to assume that our sample may well have been self-selecting towards the 'more trusting', in that those with limited or no trust would be less likely to respond. Yet, although this is an obvious limitation to the external validity of our research, the process by which most of our participants moved from negative to more positive expectations and levels of trust is, nonetheless, an instructive one for our findings.

The experiences of one female service user who was in contact with a more general community mental health team (though was generally able to manage her condition in cooperation with her GP) was in some senses an archetype of this *progress* from difficult experiences and distrust to trust. As with several of our participants, she had experienced quite negative outcomes in the past during inpatient care. The electro-convulsive therapy she had received almost 30 years before had left her with significant longer-term memory loss – particularly of her early years as a mother. While this could have impacted detrimentally on her perceptions of services, her more recent contact with one senior mental health professional in particular – a consultant psychologist – had been especially positive, as had the ongoing help from her GP.

When referring to her contact with a community mental health team, she described how this had also been tainted by some very negative experiences initially – where the professionals were too demanding and appeared highly insensitive to her current condition:

> "Yeah they were too bombastic … when you come to somebody's house and you start telling them what to do. [They] made me feel guilty that I wasn't up and washed and dressed and, you know, they were a bit of the old-fashioned type … 'Pull yourself together', which is the last thing you should say to somebody." (*Service user 4*)

This first interaction with a community team was, thus, far from trust-inspiring. In referring to being forced to go to shops and other public places that she did not feel ready for, she noted: "Bewildering … you know, frightened to death!".

Yet when these professionals were replaced, their two successors were able to generate significant levels of trust in spite of the earlier experiences. Indeed, in many senses, the negative experiences with the previous professionals made it comparatively straightforward for the new professionals to present themselves as competent and caring – such was the contrast in facework experiences for the service user. Hence, the description of why these latter professionals were seen so positively and trusted significantly suggests that these perceptions were based on relatively straightforward caring interactions and basic help around the house:

> "They made me feel confident, they *gave* me confidence [participant's emphasis]…. You know, they'd be pleased if you were washed and dressed when they came. You know, 'Oh, you've really done well'. And they'd look around things and, you know, help you put the washing…. Then I had a couple of carers at one time … and they were very good, you know, they'd come and help you do your housework … and do things."

This participant was therefore able to develop trust in spite of previous negative experiences in terms of both inpatient care and contact with a community team. This would seem to be related to the quality of the facework and direct-public experiences with the more recent professionals – where verbal and non-verbal signs combined to indicate the professionals' embeddedness in certain normative frameworks that were seen as compatible with her interests and needs (Brown et al, 2011b). Her trust was described in this context as focused very much on these individuals and their characteristics. The sharp contrast in the nature of her interactions between the negative and positive episodes emphasised the latter professionals' lack of embeddedness within the overly instrumental and demanding concerns of their predecessors. Instead, the quality of communication suggested their embeddedness within norms of patient care and this was corroborated by ongoing verbal support as well as non-verbal actions (eg assistance with housework) and gestures (Brown et al, 2011b: 289).

Thus, an empirical picture gradually emerges of how the significance of the interpersonal, due to its richness in private and direct-public experiences, is able to override more negative views of the system. Even where service users have themselves encountered poor facework and negative outcomes from treatment, these obstacles to trust at a particular time may actually make it easier for new professionals to set themselves apart as trustworthy – competent and caring – in some instances. This is more likely to be the case where the professionals are sensitive to the problems encountered by service users in the past and the difficulties they face in developing trusting relations as a result (Helene Hem et al, 2008). The importance of trusted figures within the social network of the service user (key family members and friends), and the importance of engaging these actors within the care set-up of the service user (see Piippo and Aaltonen, 2008), similarly attests to the significance of the interpersonal in developing trust.

Box 2.3: Developing trust through quality professional communication

A consultant psychiatrist participant in our research underlined the basic trust challenge that mental health services face as follows:

> "Being able to engage them. Making this person sitting in front of me – believing that it's totally ridiculous what's happening, and he shouldn't really be here – believe that there is a value of him coming to see me and maybe listening to what I say and maybe believing what I'm saying to him to some extent."

She outlined a number of ways in which such engagement could be built, with quality of relationships and communication being central to this:

> "Well, communication is key, isn't it? It's just really key, not only with the patient but with the family, with the other professionals but again – I will go to this engaging empathy sort of relationship with the patient. So yes communication obviously is….You have to work on them all the time….And I think self-reflection is very important. And also trying all the time to train yourself to not be judgemental because it's only human to be judgemental and other doctors are definitely judgemental."

In this latter sense, this professional points to one of the potentially significant features of trust that is disregarded by a number of studies of trust in healthcare (an important exception is Pilgrim et al, 2011) and that is the difficulty encountered by professionals in trusting service users or patients. Such problems may become evident within communication and, therefore, hinder the development of mutually open, trusting relationships (Maidment et al, 2011).

Other obstacles to trust, besides problematic histories with mental health services, include more straightforward interpersonal dynamics between the service user and the professional:

> "And the person themselves, yeah, their own make-up, their own beliefs ... sometimes people ... wouldn't believe a certain professional just because, you know, the way they look, their colour, something like that. And this is again only human. We've got to accept that. Yeah the age does matter, gender matters. That all matters, but on an individual basis. We cannot generalise. Yeah, so age matters, ethnicity matters, gender matters, all of that matters, but ... for some people more than others."

These interpersonal aspects could be worked around with communication skills as well as team flexibility. Overall, a working description of what trust in mental health services might resemble is this:

> "Well I think it means that they believe the services would help them and even if that does not meet their expectations 100%, they would accept that. Because obviously, you know, we're not magic ... we're not magicking things out of air. But they believe the service can help them and they believe that even the shortfalls in the service should be accounted for. They're not expecting perfection."

A further contrast to our recent research in other domains of healthcare was that the mental health professionals who participated in our research appeared especially attuned to trust as an important factor within their healthcare relationship with service users. Again, there may be aspects of self-selection occurring here (though our response rate for professionals was very high). However, that a number of professionals across the three services were so sensitive to dynamics around trust may offer further insights into how problems with trust in the past may be overcome.

Particular approaches for building trust, as emerged within our research, will be considered further in the chapters to follow. In the meantime, Box 2.3 refers to one consultant psychiatrist's account of how trust can be built even within difficult circumstances. The account presented draws attention to the underlying difficulties amidst the context of mental health services for winning trust, while also pointing towards certain sensitivities and approaches that make trust more likely. Fundamental to the account offered by this participant was the significance of communication, emphasising that this is a skill that needs to be consistently worked on, honed and reflected upon. This perspective, combined with the other data and the theoretical framework presented earlier, further underlines the significance and potency of facework (and the private experiences therein) for trust.

Conclusion

This chapter began with the acknowledgement that trust within the particular context of this study – mental health services – is problematic given a number of layers of 'experience' that bear upon the perceptions of service users. The generally negative portrayal of the capabilities and motivations of mental health services and psychiatry within the public sphere is often accompanied by a range of negative prior experiences of service users. Concerns about the efficacy of interventions and the possibility of negative side effects – either physiological, mental or social (in terms of stigma) – represent serious obstacles for individuals approaching and developing effective, trusting relationships with services.

Yet, as has been addressed both theoretically and empirically, there are a number of ways in which these apparent impediments to trust can be overcome. In many senses, the possibilities for trust, in spite of apparently good reasons against it, are rooted in the nature of trust as an active, constructed, pragmatic endeavour by which knowledge is inferred through past experiences. Drawing on Schutzian phenomenology, we have argued that three different forms of experience – mediated, public–direct and private–interactive – are relevant within this inferential process, but that private experiences are the most concrete and, therefore, relevant for trust.

Crucial to our analysis, however, is the notion that all three forms are significant and influential upon one another. Mediated experiences, for example, are significant in directing attention towards certain concerns and facets of professional interactions or institutional practices (Schutz, 1972: 196) that might otherwise remain unnoticed. Meanwhile, we also argued that effective interpersonal communicative action may be significant in developing shared understandings that lead to improved direct–public experiences, such as more accurate prescribing. Improvements in these more direct, tangible experiences may in turn undergird future interpretations of interaction as signifying benevolent motives and competence.

Thus, we have proposed a model of knowledge formation within trust in terms of a trialectic between the three different formats of experience. This model was initially developed within a quite different trust context (gynaecological oncology; see Brown, 2009a), yet we have argued here that this trialectic is useful in explaining the general primacy of facework for trust within mental health settings. The phenomenological framework on which this model is based is also insightful in underlining the *active* manner through which significant negative direct experiences (diagnostic or treatment failings) are able to be bracketed off to the extent that general positive assumptions towards the system and/or positive interactive experiences enable this.

Notes

[1] It is important to recognise that *institution* is a very fluid term within the social sciences, especially in sociology. In the sociological literature, institution often refers to patterned

or structured forms of action across a particular social group or society. Within more general parlance institution refers to particular 'bodies' or organisations within society. The term is applied in this study to refer to a hybrid of these two different aspects – in this sense the way in which normative frameworks across society are visible through the formation, existence and outworking of particular organisations or bodies of people (for example professions). This is significant in that perceptions of a particular organisation are partly related to its own distinct characteristics, personnel and performance, but are also influenced by the normative structures it represents and embodies (Brown and Flores, 2011).

[2] Although, more recently, Approved Social Workers can also initiate the sectioning of a service user by which s/he is admitted to inpatient care against his or her will, current laws still require the assessment of a psychiatrist who, in some senses, has the final world, albeit within an interdisciplinary process.

[3] Dentistry might be another quite different, but similarly culturally burdened, area of healthcare that renders trust problematic.

[4] Corrigan and Watson (2002) underline the range of experiences and responses to potential stigma of serious mental illness – in this sense, it is imperative to avoid simplistic notions of a general response.

[5] As apparent within our very small sample of service users (eight participants), responses suggested that those with a diagnosis of bipolar experienced this label as less a form of 'spoiled identity' (Goffman, 1963) than those diagnosed as schizophrenic. This may potentially be related to recent generally sympathetic depictions in the public sphere (eg the character 'Stacey Slater' in the popular BBC soap opera *EastEnders*), or even positive ones (eg the highly regarded and respected actor and television/Twitter personality Stephen Fry who has been very candid about his experiences of bipolar disorder). Various participants referred to these two 'characters' as helping themselves and others understand and normalise the condition. This was not the case for schizophrenia, which, from a Parsonian perspective, can be seen as being portrayed as less compatible with the functionalist demands of modern society.

[6] In addressing the relevance of mammography screening to trust, Solbjør (2008) explores an interesting liminal area between these mediated and the direct formats of experience. On the one hand, technology is used as a medium of making the body visible, yet that this is a direct means by which the service user is able to view her own body renders it closer to the 'direct-experience' format discussed in this chapter. Certainly, there would seem to be much potency attached to these images in considerations of trust.

[7] Some of the aspects of the 'private experiences', as they are conceived by individuals in relation to their experiences of healthcare, resonate with the processes by which 'common-sense' ideas of health become real for people within social contexts, as explored by Cornwell (1985).

[8] After all, it is only another being, rather than mere notions, that can help us solve the problem of complexity (Luhmann, 1979); or, to put it another way, there are certain

matters in life 'about which we prefer to think in absolutes. We delegate the relative way of thinking to another, who becomes our agent. He runs our risks for us. We like to believe him endowed with charisma' (Cherrington Hughes, 1994: 81). It is within private experiences that we find this other and interact with him or her to establish these qualities.

[9] Hence, what some social scientists distinguish through reference to trust (in motives) and confidence (in competence) is a problematic dualism. While analytically neat, such a distinction is not reflective of the understandings of many participants in our study and, indeed, other research (eg Calnan and Rowe, 2008).

[10] This was the only one of our eight service user informants to have become an inpatient via the criminal justice system. A study of the experiences of inpatients within medium secure units found that this was the most common route for patients (Riordan and Humphreys, 2007) and this route of 'referral' is likely to imbue services with negative connotations for these patients.

[11] Here, there is a stark contrast with the experiences of the interval breast cancer patients interviewed by Solbjør and colleagues (2010). These patients had largely positive experiences and were, therefore, seemingly able to bracket away a negative experience as an exception to the rule – albeit a very significant exception. The ongoing negative experiences described by the mental health service user quoted here means that any potential bracketing away would require too great a 'leap of faith' to make trust possible. Negative experiences were the rule.

THREE

Bridging uncertainty by constructing trust: the rationality of *irrational* approaches

Chapter Two analysed various ways in which service users developed trust in spite of general public perceptions, not to mention significant personal experiences, which might have warded against such positive expectations.[1] Many of the social contexts and professional relations described by participants suggested positive grounds for trust, yet histories of negative outcomes combined with the multiple uncertainties described towards the end of Chapter One (regarding the possibility and durability of recovery, the effectiveness of interventions, and the professionals' embedding within a risk-prioritised service) point towards an apparent *unknowableness* associated with mental healthcare or, indeed, healthcare in general (Titmuss, 2004). As a recent study makes clear, inherent to healthcare are uncertainties pertaining to the range of possible outcomes, more positive or negative in their nature: 'At its best, healthcare will be a testimony to our capacity to be interdependent. At its worst, it will mistreat, maim and kill us' (Pilgrim et al, 2011: 59). Acting within positive expectations for the future amidst such manifold uncertainties – Titmuss (2004: 173) lists 'thirteen characteristics [which] are indicative of the many subtle aspects of uncertainty and unpredictability which pervade modern medical care systems' – would appear to require a 'suspension of belief' or 'leap of faith' (Möllering, 2001), which transcends rational thought or consideration.

Preceding chapters have touched upon at least three features of trust that would *prima facie* seem to underline this 'less-than-rational' status (Williamson, 1993) – or what Zinn (2008a) refers to as trust's position 'in between' the rational and non-rational. First, the way service users (and, indeed, professionals) focused particularly on the 'presentation of self' – or facework – for appraising the trustworthiness of another would seem to be a highly tentative, subjectively constructed and far from robust means of building reliable knowledge about another. Recent debacles within the English NHS underline the 'dark side' of trust (Davies and Mannion, 2000) – where a highly esteemed family doctor was able to kill hundreds of patients or where a prestigious regional centre for surgery had an abnormally high surgical mortality rate for infants (Pilgrim et al, 2011: 131–45). Impressions, not least adeptly managed facework, can be utterly misleading, and, therefore, the gap between perceptions (trust) and substance (trustworthiness) becomes a problematic one (O'Neill, 2002). Experiences of service users and professionals who had all been let down, in various ways, in the past underlines this *liability* of a trust that is strongly contingent on interaction.

Second, not only is a partial or total reliance on facework an apparently flimsy basis for making oneself vulnerable to a professional or institution (or patient in the professionals' case), but, moreover, the emotional component that is inherent to this format of processing information within interactions (or forms of knowledge derived from other sources) might also be described as crude – a source of bias that wards against a more thorough processing of salient information (eg Tiedens and Linton, 2001).[2] Third, we also noted examples in the last chapter where bad experiences, which could feasibly reoccur in the future, were 'bracketed away'. A phenomenological framework for considering trust emphasised that decision-making processes involved participants almost wilfully focusing upon certain experiences and disregarding others (Brown, 2009a). From this perspective, trust begins to resemble a form of cognitive dissonance or 'aintegrative thinking' (Lomranz and Benyamini, 2009), which, when combined with its interpersonal preoccupation and emotionality, appears as a profoundly less-than-rational or even irrational project.

The critical approach to trust outlined in the preceding paragraphs is written from a narrow (and somewhat caricatured) 'rational actor' perspective. The remainder of this chapter will proceed to develop a critique of this standpoint and, in particular, will problematise the constricted conception of *rationality* applied in the various branches of social science that adopt such a position. Rather than positing the interpersonal, affective and bracketing bases of trust as aspects of irrational behaviour, these approaches to managing and constructing knowledge amidst uncertainty will be seen as necessary, appropriate and often highly effective.

Moreover, the analysis presented in the chapter will seek to move beyond straightforward and problematic considerations of rational–irrational or rational–non-rational dualisms (Brown, 2009b). Zinn's (2008a) spectrum – from the rational-calculative (ie risk-oriented) towards the 'non-rational' (hope and faith) – is useful in the way it can be interpreted as representing a range of different processes by which the limits of knowing (and thus the intractable problem of uncertainty) are less (risk) or more explicitly (hope) recognised. Nevertheless, the chapter begins by suggesting that ascriptions of rationality are problematic at a logical-philosophical level (in that they tend ultimately towards tautological – self-referential – forms of reasoning). Connected to this critique is the concern that, from the perspective of effective social-scientific analysis, rationality represents an explanatory cul-de-sac; one where labels of irrationality merely distract from complex explanations of socially embedded action.

Rationality as an obstacle to social analysis

One of the great strengths of a number of current research programmes that reflect upon the concept of trust is their interdisciplinarity. As observed in the earlier chapters of this volume, transaction cost economics (eg Williamson, 1993), political science (eg Dunn, 1993) and a range of other perspectives (from psychology to ethics; for a useful synthesis, see Pilgrim et al, 2011) offer a broad range of valuable insights that shed significant light on the process of trust and various factors that are causally related. Within the domain of sociology, a number of studies into trust emerge from a broader stream of research into how individuals and organisations cope within contexts of apparent 'risk and uncertainty'. This field is very much influenced by economics, cognitive psychology and broader policy research and, as a result, contains a number of 'rational actor' frames and 'expert/lay' distinctions more or less implicitly assumed within its analyses. These begin with neat conceptions of scientifically informed and appropriate behaviour, and lay tendencies towards dysfunctional or irrational behaviour (Thaler and Sunstein's [2008] book *Nudge* is a current, often insightful, archetype of this position), and often seek to understand the grounds of irrationality as a way of benefiting from such tendencies (eg on stock markets, see Hirschey and Nofsinger, 2009) or in working to correct/mitigate them (Thaler and Sunstein, 2008).

These analytical approaches, when applied to research into trust (social policy-oriented and more general social-scientific), thus tend to be mistrustful of trust (Ashraf et al, 2003). Studies often note the way in which social contexts of trust and confidence act to warp the rational policymaking process and, therefore, the ability of experts to guide lay people towards a safer, more efficient, more enlightened future. They also tend to emphasise the non-calculative aspects of trust (contrasting them to the more formal modelling of risk) – where this lack of calculation is held up as problematic; a source of bias and, thus, ultimately irrational.

Of course, these ascriptions of irrationality, or a lack of rationality, are laden with a vast array of assumptions. These relate most profoundly to the ability of calculative models to effectively cope with and overcome uncertainty (Gray, 2009a) and are rooted within an Enlightenment paradigm that privileges certain notions of knowledge formation, processing and application over others. Gray (2009b) points to the weak foundations of such assumptions (outlining the key tenets of this 'positivist catechism'), and it is in this self-referential hierarchy of knowledge formats that the tautological nature of ascriptions of 'rationality' becomes clearer.

The grounds on which rationality–irrationality distinctions are made in relation to trust are normative due to the extent to which there is an idealised notion of science that is incorrectly assumed to be effective for dealing with future uncertainty (Gray, 2009a). The hegemonic position of a particular format of scientific reasoning makes possible the elevation of generalisable knowledge (Habermas, 1971; Adorno and Horkheimer, 1973) and a corresponding depriviledging and debasement of (socialised) subjectivity and personal experience (O'Neill, 1995). Yet the application of rationality in understanding individual decisions, which Weber suggests is possible in a 'morally neutral' manner (Brubaker, 1984: 94), is at odds with the meaning-based, substantive rationality by which decisions fit into the evolving format of personal norms and values within the wider life-course (Weber, 1975 [1904]) – with analyses becoming unavoidably 'morally charged' in this latter sense (Brubaker, 1984: 94). The array of different goals and consequences that are meaningful to individuals, in terms of their choice of ends and, moreover, preferences for certain methods of decision-making, entail that critiques in terms of rationality are difficult to substantiate other than through value-laden conceptions of what is 'appropriate'. In this manner, appraisals of rationality become self-referential and thus err towards the tautological (Brown, 2009b).

Even if goals and preferences are set to one side, and we focus purely on the rationality of *process*, clear distinctions between the rational and non-rational become difficult to uphold due to a lack of existing examples of decision-making in any social context that can be deemed *fully* rational. Given that everyday human behaviour meets the criteria of being 'reasonable' and 'deliberative', and that the ideal-type of rational action is 'so idealised that it cannot be found anywhere in the world' (O'Neill, 1995: 181; see also Keynes, 1936), it seems that the only aspect that sets 'lay' behaviour apart from its generalisably 'rational' counterpoint is the former's causal complexity.

From this basic starting point, an argument develops that to label behaviour or decision-making as irrational is not only difficult to substantiate, but, moreover, obscures and distracts from the salience of context – both socio-biographical and immediate – and the deep ways in which decision-making is embedded therein. This is the main deficiency as far as effective social analysis is concerned, in the sense that tautology can be viewed as an intellectual *cul-de-sac* that blocks deeper and broader understanding. In avoiding these problematic and limiting distinctions or categorisations, the rest of the chapter pursues deeper understandings of the inherent rationality of trusting – based on a misquotation of Waugh (1945) that 'to understand all is to consider all as rational' (Brown, 2009b: 10).

Trust as necessary, appropriate and effective

The utility of facework as an approach to coping amidst heightened uncertainty and vulnerability

In the previous chapter, we discussed the concreteness of interpersonal facework in contrast to more abstract notions, and the former's relative significance for trust. In this subsection, we develop somewhat further these understandings of the utility and efficacy of interpersonal communication as a basis for trust. Drawing on literature beyond phenomenology, we emphasise the extent to which a predominant role for facework within processes of trust is necessary, appropriate and effective. Thus we stress the inherent *reasonableness* of trusting through this format of knowledge.

In acknowledging the extent to which prescriptions of rational behaviour (at the organisational or individual level) are detached from the realities of decision-making and, thus, problematic, Herbert Simon (1982) develops his notion of 'bounded rationality', which emphasises the extent to which all decisions are inherently focused on certain concerns and, thus, disregard (or are blind towards) others. This model of boundedness is forced upon actors making decisions due to their limited abilities and time to consider a wider or complete range of alternatives. An early example of such an alternative model of limited or bounded decision-making is that labelled by Lindblom (1959: 79) as 'disjointed incrementalism'. In critiquing fanciful notions regarding the possibility of root-and-branch reviews within the policymaking process as a fully rational consideration, he asserts that this 'is of course impossible. It assumes intellectual capacities and sources of information that men simply do not possess'. Lindblom (1959: 79) goes on to note how policymakers 'restrict their attention to relatively few values and relatively few alternative policies'.

Individual actors are, in many senses, similarly bounded in their decisions by necessity and practicality. If we consider the narrow model of 'rationality' invoked within some domains of social science as 'a thought process or a decision where one is fully aware of the different options and takes an active part in taking the decision or in developing a plan of action' (Pilgrim et al, 2011: 201), then we can also conclude that this is unattainable. Instead, the complexity and uncertainty that are a feature of modern society (see Introduction) are managed in various formats of boundedness through 'a course of action that is satisfactory or – "good enough"' (Simon, 1976: xxix).

Trust is precisely one such strategy that is necessary, good enough and, thus, appropriate in managing complexity and uncertainty in particular contexts (Luhmann, 1979; Petit, 1995). In contrast to calculative models that are misleading in their pretence to 'deal' with future uncertainty (Gray, 2009a), trust continues to recognise uncertainty and the possibility for negative outcomes. Yet, whereas a proper recognition of uncertainty from a fully calculative position would engender 'paralysis' (Luhmann, 1979) due to the very limits of calculation, trust can be understood as effective insofar as it enables action in the midst of uncertainty – while not acting blindly to the possibility of being let down (Calnan and Rowe, 2008).[3]

The trust that emerges through interpersonal communication is especially suited to developing these more qualified forms of expectations through its enhanced ability to establish and verify knowledge through communicative action. In this manner, facework:

> is doubly important, not simply in fostering a familiar and relational scenario but also one where the patient can be convinced of the competence of the professional through communication of his/her interests and the corresponding assurance by the professional that these are congruent with the proposed intervention. In this sense trust can be seen as communicative in the way it is 'doubly contingent' on the 'interpretive accomplishments' of both actors (Habermas 1987, p 262). For how can a patient be assured that his/her best interests are central if they have not had adequate opportunity to convey these interests and voice their concerns? (Brown, 2009a: 393)

While 'compatibility of interests' and 'competence' may normally be thought of as two quite distinct notions within trust, these twin pillars often become intertwined within the communicative interactions between service users and professionals (Calnan and Rowe, 2008; Pilgrim et al, 2011). Here, one service user notes how the mode of interactions, his involvement within these and the thoroughness in the professional's conduct combine to form a trustworthy professional:

> "I think [my more recent care coordinator] talks more openly about options, the options I have, the avenues we can explore. I don't really think I had that before. She seemed to be more, dare I say, more scientific in her approach, she seemed to say 'Well, we'll do … we'll do this….'
>
> … she's got it [a certain quality]. She does it…. She does things in the right way. She conducts herself properly. She does things thoroughly and I think that's obvious from what she's done and from her work behind the scenes and where she's got me [to] now." (*Service user 6*)

In this instance, thoroughness is both a sign of having the service user's interests at heart as well as a professionalism associated with competence:

> "Enthusiasm I think. A caring but professional attitude. Trust. Trust is so important. I think that's why I kind of wanted to get involved in it [participating in the research] really. I think if you think of yourself when you go to a health professional in any way if you don't trust them you can't possibly…. It makes everything a nonsense really, doesn't it?"

> "Yeah. It's about the fact that I'm here actually to assist them and I see that as being the best way of actually making them feel they're in safe hands if that makes sense." (*Social worker*)

From this professional perspective, there is a similar recognition that an enthusiasm or readiness to assist reassures a vulnerable service user that they are in safe (competent) hands.

The combining of expertise with helpfulness is perhaps most usefully captured in the Aristotelian notion of virtue, which Pilgrim and colleagues (2011: 66) note as the bringing together of 'the efficacy of carrying out that role as skilfully as possible and the character traits associated with such an achievement'. Ascertaining the presence of this 'practical wisdom' ('*phronēsis*') (Pilgrim et al, 2011: 66) is beyond the calculable, for this would only result in fractured focusing on the generalisable aspects of this craftwork (Sennett, 2008) to the ignorance of the tacit knowledge and the attentiveness bound up with this.

Emotion as a reasonable basis for decision-making

A further Aristotelian insight gleamed through the work of Pilgrim and colleagues (2011: 63) is the 'integration of reason and emotion in a holistic and naturalistic view of a human being'. The partiality towards the calculative within certain 'rational actor' approaches noted earlier entails that emotions are often seen as having a deceiving or skewing effect on decisions; where an ideal judgement context involves such 'animal spirits' being minimised, offset or worked around (Akerlof and Shiller, 2009). Once again, this deprivileging of an intrinsic part of everyday action (for 'expert' and 'lay' person alike) is rooted in a deeper social history of science – one where emotions have often been connected to the body, and, as such, have typically been seen within domains such as social psychology (among many) as 'unbidden and uncontrollable' (Hochschild, 1979: 551), within the paradigmatic setting of a deeper Cartesian dualism.

If we look to step beyond this prejudice towards the emotionality of decision-making, then we see that the emotions present within trust decisions – as with the communicative facets of trust – are necessary (and inherent), appropriate (in their appraisal of a holistic notion of virtue) and an effective and efficient heuristic. We have noted elsewhere that communication provides a more nuanced understanding of the necessary blend of competence and care that enables quality service provision, and which calculative checking mechanisms are blind to (Nettleton et al, 2008; Brown and Calnan, 2010). Emotions are similarly vital for this verificatory process regarding virtue to be enacted (Pilgrim et al, 2011).

A growing literature within social analyses of action amidst uncertainty, often influenced by Keynes (1936), acknowledges the inevitable and vital role played by emotions within decision-making (eg Pixley, 2004; Zinn, 2008a). 'Current research in neuroscience, cognitive psychology, behavioural economics, and sociology indicates that emotions may provide an effective basis for making decisions about risk and managing uncertainty' (Zinn, 2008a: 445). While many studies of trust tend to refer to emotions as an alternative to, or working in tandem with, knowledge in a more cognitive sense, other more recent work emphasises the heuristic or intuitive role of emotions – the way these provide quickly accessible reactions amidst uncertainty, which relate to, are shaped by and draw upon past experiences (Brown, 2009a) – and the salience of emotions in facilitating 'choice of strategy' (Barbalet, 2009: 374). Furthermore:

> if emotions underscore values, interests and meanings in social life, then they are implicated in rational as well as irrational conduct and outlook, and the distinction between rational action and emotional action loses its relevance when emotion is seen to underlie all action. (Barbalet, 2009: 9)

In this light, it can be argued that emotions are efficient heuristics in themselves (Gigerenzer and Todd, 1999) – facilitating judgements and providing 'fast and frugal' (Gigerenzer and Todd, 1999) modes for drawing on past experiences and applying this *knowledge* to situations where there is a paucity of information in its more generalisable format. The innate unknowableness of the future makes apparent the impossibility of calculation in an inductive format (Möllering, 2001); hence, why apparently unfavourable comparisons with formal rationality, as a means of critiquing the approach of trust, are argued here to be inappropriate or even misguided. Trust is not, then, 'resorted to' due to limitations of knowledge processing on the part of the truster, but becomes relevant and often necessary due to the *impossibility* of knowing – which is a feature of the actor's future orientation (Keynes, 1936; Barbalet, 2009).

Barbalet proceeds to refer to a number of the ways in which emotions are useful in binding together different processes that must be reconciled for trust to be enacted, but which are, nonetheless, difficult or impossible to achieve without the 'intelligence of emotions' (Nussbaum, 2001). One example of this is what Barbalet refers to as the double-hermeneutic involved in trust, by which certain qualities of the trustee are considered on the one hand, and need to be reconciled with another set of concerns of the truster in light of his or her own context:

> An essential feature of all emotions, including the emotional basis of trust, is a process of double non-deliberative appraisal. These are: appraisal of the object of the emotion, what it means to the emoting subject; and also, appraisal of the subject's own needs, capacities, and possible action strategies or responses in relation to the object. (Barbalet, 2009: 282)

Similar to the way in which communication directly enables expressions of the truster's needs and their comparison with the motives and claims of the trustee, emotions thus assist judgements by which the 'purchase' (or goal) of trust and the likelihood of its realisation – to 'create an outcome otherwise unavailable' – is appraised in the light of the 'cost' involved (Barbalet, 2009: 367). This cost is essentially one of dependency (Barbalet, 2009: 367) and is discussed in detail in Chapter Four.

Further assessments are also required such as evaluating the 'self-trust' of the truster and, thus, his or her ability to accurately gauge the potential trustee and their situation. Reconciling these three discrete notions is highly complex and/or problematic, yet is achievable through the affective capacities of social actors. The ability of an emotional reaction to quickly reconcile a number of multifarious considerations as well as bridging over the uncertainty of outcomes is visible in the following example. Here, one service user, who had not felt able to trust any mental health professionals sufficiently to talk openly with them, describes (several years later) the first encounter with two social workers who she felt she *could* trust:

> *Service user 8:* "I still remember. I remember both of them, one male, one female, just kind of sat down with me and listened and just really

took me seriously and … I mean even just thinking about it makes me breathe more easily. It just … I only saw them once!"

Interviewer: "Would you say you had a lot of trust or a lot of kind of …"

Service user 8: "Yeah. Just almost instantaneous with them."

Interviewer: "Sure. And was there anything in particular about them or is that hard to put your finger on?"

Service user 8: "I remember they smiled. I remember that I didn't feel like a patient and that seemed to be a quite clear distinction actually between the psychiatry place and going in to the … because it [where you waited at the 'psychiatry place'] felt like a waiting room whereas at the social work place somehow it really just didn't … it felt more like you were going into a set of offices … and I suppose my anticipation was that I would be de-medicalised if you like because it was a social work … a social worker."

Emotions and their role in the social world are an epistemological challenge to the researcher due to their partial existence beyond the bounds of subjective awareness, yet this excerpt points towards the apparent emotional departure point for this brief, yet highly trusting, relationship. The way in which an instantaneous emotional reaction brought together numerous different considerations – both those expressed here and, we might presume, others not expressed (such as those pertaining to self-trust) – suggests the integrating role that emotions perform.

The excerpt refers, furthermore, to other components that are salient for trust as features of emotional appraisal – not least the body and space. The emotions relating to trust in these two social workers elicits a physical response even as this is recounted several years later and make apparent how bodily sensation can act as a form of tacit knowledge and, thus, trust (Parr and Davidson, 2008; Brown et al, 2011b). Meanwhile, as was referred to by a number of service user and professional participants, the spatial surroundings were also significant for trust. From some perspectives (eg a narrow 'rational actor' approach), the appearance of the building would seem irrelevant to the trustworthiness of an individual practitioner and the delivery of instrumental outcomes of healthcare. Yet through the affective understandings of space, an individual is able to relate a current setting to prior experiences within certain socio-physical environments and the likelihood of positive outcomes. Here, the non-medical 'feel' of the space is complexly bound up with the possibility of a less medicalised format of help, as well as reducing the experience of stigma associated with more overtly 'psychiatric' institutional settings. Woven together, the different characteristics of this spatial context are, thus, held to be conducive to trust.

Subjective constructions and bracketing away

The preceding section noted how the unknowables inherent to future-oriented social contexts raise at least two clear problems. First, the number of different considerations that need to be reconciled for trust to be possible highlights what might be called the *integration problematic*. This includes the profound difficulties of making multiple evaluations – of systems, of trustees embedded within these institutions, of one's personal context and needs, and of trust in one's own appraisals – and, moreover, of relating these to one another, given that there are few common terms of reference between them. Second, we noted earlier that the basic epistemic issues referred to by a number of studies emphasise that the future-oriented nature of the uncertainty encountered is not just a challenge to formal rationality, but an unassailable monolith – 'we simply do not know' (Gray, 2009a: 13).

Following Barbalet (2009), among others, we concluded that narrow, formal/procedural conceptions of rationality are unable to cope with trust – either as a tool for considering who to trust or as a basis for analysing trust. In contrast, a more broadly conceived, substantive notion of rationality is highly relevant and, indeed, useful in describing how the application of communicative action and emotional appraisal are highly rational in their overcoming of these features of the unknowable. The notion of a 'forced option' (Barbalet, 2009: 372 [following William James]) is instructive here in underlining that acting outside of calculative formats is necessary and efficient in bringing about a situation that would otherwise be inaccessible:

> In this sense the employment of 'a trustful and not necessarily practical attitude' (Vaitkus 1990, p 287) may be a highly rational action within the 'game' of interpretation (Vaitkus 1991) where the intended goal is the minimisation of anxiety in the face of extreme vulnerability and lack of alternatives. (Brown, 2009: 401)

Trust, from this perspective, is an inherently rational component within the coping strategies of service users and professionals, but is also, as we have argued elsewhere, inherent to the nature of 'scientific' decision-making, which would be incapable of advancing or generalising were it not for such trust-oriented processes of bracketing away (Brown and Calnan, forthcoming). In the same manner by which a rational-scientific-bureaucratic process – in our article, NICE appraisals of new drugs in terms of their cost-effectiveness (Brown and Calnan, forthcoming) – would be unable to reach a decision were the actors involved not able to 'assume away' various uncertainties, the processes described here by which professionals and service users bracket away uncertainty through emotion-based and communicative-oriented trust is equally appropriate as part of a 'modified "substantive" rationality (without regard to values) that connects actor with outcome' (Barbalet, 2009: 382).

The problem of the unknowable future was referred to by service users and especially professionals:

> "Yes.... It's very difficult as well because, I mean, I know we've got clients who will only tell us what they want us to know and … something might happen and you think, 'oh gosh there's a whole different side to them that we don't know about because they just won't let us in to that'." (*Community psychiatric nurse [CPN]*)

The impossibility of fully knowing and understanding the service users with which they work means that for another CPN trust is at once difficult and yet indispensable:

> *CPN*: "Yeah. I think you've got to work together, you know, to get an end result really. Yeah. If you're kind of … you know, if they haven't got any trust in you it's … I don't think it's really gonna work properly, you know, so you're giving more."
>
> *Interviewer*: "What about you trusting in them?"
>
> *CPN*: "Yeah. You have to as well. You have to in some ways."

This 'forced choice', although a complicating issue where choice is intrinsic to trust (Luhmann, 1979),[4] is also testament to the inherent rationality of trusting even where this might be difficult (Petit, 1995). By its very nature, trust is not straightforward, and yet the possibilities for future outcomes that are opened up through trust entail that it continues to be pursued and conceived as a viable, vital option:

> "Well I think my belief is that I trust my patients. I have got no reason to distrust them.… And I will find the reason for them if they don't take their medication. And often, if you show them the trust, they will come back and show you the same, you know?
>
> It's difficult to make a social judgement that your patient is not telling you the truth but even so – if you felt that they were *unable* rather than not telling you the truth – unable to say what they wanted to say – you give them the time to allow them to give you the full story." (*Psychiatrist*) [participant's emphasis]

This account rationalises reasons for trusting service users on the basis of a lack of evidence to the contrary, as well as the reciprocal benefits of trusting. The second paragraph, which explains away that which might otherwise be considered a reason not to trust, is highly sympathetic. Some practitioners might argue that this approach is naive, and yet it enables a continuation of trust (as opposed to checking) even in the face of disappointments. Moreover, this perspective ensures that communicative paths are pursued, where otherwise a more restrictive mode of seeking control would hamper interaction and would, thus, undermine trust further in the longer term.

Dispositions and forming knowledge of others: *habitus* and trust

Taken together, the three subsections of the preceding section emphasise the extent to which trust is profoundly social, phenomenological and rooted in past experiences. The construction of knowledge through communication, involving the interpretation of verbal and non-verbal signs, relies upon interpretive schemas that are fashioned through previous social contexts and interactions. The meaning attached to certain signs and the way these are deciphered as denoting a particular 'latent intentionality' (Merleau-Ponty, 1968: 213) are made possible by past experiences and wider socio-cultural norms that 'teach' (and thus facilitate) such interpretation. Similarly, we have noted examples where emotions can, in many senses, be seen as drawing upon past experiences and relating these, through affective experiences,[5] to the decision-making in the present.

Thus, an argument can be further developed regarding the way quite specific social contexts, and the socio-biographies that emerge therein, may bear significantly on people's overall tendencies towards trusting. Where negative outcomes and disappointments have been a common experience, a wider array of signs and contexts are likely to be interpreted as indicating the likelihood of problematic future outcomes. Similarly, emotional reactions within certain settings may tend towards distrust or even mistrust where these dispositions have been inculcated through the common occurrence of negative incidents, experiences of deceit or where an inconsistency between signs and outcomes makes inferential understandings less reliable and, thus, problematic to apply.

Box 3.1: Dispositions towards distrust – views of professionals

Almost all the professionals we interviewed referred to difficulties encountered in developing trusting relations with a certain number of the service users within their current or recent caseload. Often, this was referred to as rooted in a number of past experiences of service users:

"Yeah, if I take that into account ... and I'm thinking about a lot of people I'm working with at the moment who have experienced a lot of ... or had a lot of experience in their life where trust isn't there, or they've put trust in people and it's been broken, or they've felt betrayed in some way, or they've got lots of faith and hope ... that somebody will do something and then it doesn't get done. I think I keep that in mind that that's the case, so I wouldn't automatically assume that someone's going to trust me to do whatever really. So I think that might be ... working around that and keeping that in mind ... especially if things are moving a bit slower with some people [in terms of building rapport and trust]." (CPN)

Similarly, a CPN working in another service also noted the difficulty encountered when working with some service users due to a lack of trust, describing the origins of these dispositions as follows:

"It could be because, you know, a lot of them there's a lot of events that have happened whilst growing up, you know? Sexual abuse, you know, things like that really and, yeah, I'd guess that would be a big, big factor." (CPN)

The fateful moments (Giddens, 1991) referred to here can be defining in their impact on the narratives of self, and one's relating of self to others, and, consequently, a range of dispositions that an actor comes to adopt within social contexts. These dispositions are seen here by professionals to bear decisively on trust and distrust.

This background framework of trust through communicative action and emotions enables us to offer a further nuanced account of Misztal's (1996) relating of trust to the Bourdieuian concept of *habitus* (for a useful overview of Misztal's framework, see also Scambler and Britten, 2001). By understanding the way in which dispositions are inculcated within norms of interpretation, affect and associated expectations, analytical depth is added when considering certain attitudinal positions that might be described by some as 'highly trusting' – for example, the consultant quoted at the end of the preceding section. Alternatively, an individual's social biography within particular fields – within which knowledge is derived from past experiences as applied through inculcated dispositions – may create a decidedly less trusting, or mistrustful, *habitus*, which might be related by some to *paranoia*, for example, the patient who describes how "Personally, I've never been able to trust anyone as far as I can throw them" (*service user 1*).

This service user had a diagnosis of paranoid schizophrenia,[6] one that he disputed. In our role as social scientists, we have also been resistant to this and other diagnostic labels for two reasons: first, following a critical realist position towards mental illness as described by Pilgrim and Benthall (1999), we conceptualise diagnoses as one 'map' by which certain people seek to make sense of, analogise or navigate a reality (for a critical approach to diagnosis that notes their socially constructed and political function, see Moncrieff, 2010); second, to describe trust dispositions in terms of actors' diagnoses risks a further intellectual cul-de-sac. Explanations of dispositions in terms of 'psychiatric condition' and/or neurology potentially limit or distract from a deeper understanding via the salience of the social contexts within which these originate.

One relevant perspective upon the forming of trust dispositions is the work of Pilgrim and colleagues (2011: 48), who bring together a range of insights from psychoanalysis, childhood environments and developmental psychology in noting how 'the failure of trust in childhood has several implications for the roles of patients and professionals'. As these and other authors underline, it is important not to fall into the assumption that childhood experiences are *defining*, and, indeed, this should be argued for trust. But, nevertheless, the family context and other early social settings may be particularly powerful fields for inculcating dispositions towards self and others that bear upon trust in the future.

Considerations of 'early maladaptive schemas' represent a further format of conceptualising early experiences in a child's relation to self and the social environment and how these may, through 'memories, emotions, cognitions and bodily sensations' (Young et al, 2003: 61), impact upon, and thus be reinforced by, later experiences across the life-course. While this framework may be especially useful in considering behaviours labelled as personality disorders (Young et al, 2003), we argue that the dispositions of all actors, in terms of their interactions and expectations, are inculcated through prior experiences – functioning through these aspects of memory, emotion, cognition and the embodied social experience. These latter four aspects are, of course, also significantly shaped by current and more recent adult fields of social interactions and the norms functioning therein (eg Shilling and Mellor, 2007). We briefly explore some of the accounts of these dispositions in Boxes 3.1 and 3.2 as they appeared within participant narratives. While these focus predominantly upon the socially shaped *habitus* of service users, it is, of course, vital to remember that the (more or less trusting) dispositions of professionals are also significantly shaped by recent occupational, and indeed earlier, fields of social experience (Pilgrim et al, 2011).

Box 3.2: A resilient trusting *habitus* (in spite of negative experiences)

We have referred to service user 4 before (in Chapter Two) in terms of her negative experiences, and yet as an example of a service user who described very high levels of trust in spite of this. While some service users referred to a generally negative attitude towards services, with certain professionals standing out as exceptions, this particular participant referred to a positive view of services and professionals overall. The excerpt begins with brief references to her experiences of electroconvulsive therapy (ECT) before going on to refer to her continuing trust. She appears to note that this attitude might seem unlikely, given her experiences, but goes on to relate this to a *habitus* developed within an ongoing life experience of typically positive outcomes:

Service user 4: "I wasn't really in a position [to trust or not], I think half the time. You know, it wasn't very nice. I used to hate having it [ECT], you know."

Interviewer: "And did that affect how you kind of saw, for example, the doctors that were administering it…?"

Service user 4: "I just really trusted … I suppose I trusted them a lot. I didn't have a lot of problems with them. And as I say, some of the nurses were really nice. I think perhaps I was just one of the lucky ones. But I'm not a great one … I've never been a great one really for complaining … I used to just accept things because I've always been very lucky."

Interviewer: "So because you've had …"

Service user 4: "My life was always lucky. I mean we never had any money as kids but it was a great life."

Interviewer: "Things always worked out well."

Service user 4: "So.…Yeah."

Interviewer: "So do you think that's just sort of fed in. So you thought these people must be here to help me kind of thing …"

Service user 4: "Yeah. Yeah.… Even, you know, people moan about my doctor. One said, oh, she said, you know, 'I wouldn't go to him', but he's fantastic I find. So I think half the time it's how you are with other people – how they react to you."

This excerpt finishes by touching upon the way in which dispositions for relating to others have an impact on the form of relationship that develops and, moreover, the inter-subjective experience of that relationship. These patterns and expectations for interacting can, thus, continue to shape and reinforce the earlier dispositions, further inculcating these schemas over time (Young et al, 2003).

Conclusion

We began this chapter by noting the predominance of a relatively narrow, rational actor model for social-scientific considerations of how people act amidst future uncertainty. We then suggested a number of problems inherent to this approach, with regards to its *accuracy* in describing what people do, as well as the *efficacy* of procedural considerations of rationality. Correspondingly, these narrow prescriptions for assessing what is 'rational' were seen as dangerous for social research in that they deprivilege and dismiss the actions of lay people in comparison to a calculative ideal that is false and unattainable (Gray, 2009a). More significantly, the labels of 'irrationality' distract from effective social science as they focus researchers on the immediate sources of 'bias', rather than enabling a deeper account of all human action as profoundly embedded within the social.

The failure of this narrow rationality and the problems of this normative rational–irrational distinction informed the basis of the framework developed later in the chapter. We have sought to deem all accounts of trust as rational and where initial impressions might have pointed to the *irrational*, we have interpreted this rather as an indication of limited understanding on our part and of the need to further explore the socio-biographical contexts and, moreover, the very nature of formats of knowledge application within the social, which the accounts reflect.

In light of this approach, subsections within this chapter have sought to underline the profound rationality of developing trust through communicative and affective experiences and interaction. By building on a range of literature that overcomes the dualisms between mind and body, cognition and affect, it becomes clear that embodied communicative interactions and the emotions that reflect these are necessary, appropriate and efficient bases of trust. Indeed, given the intractable problem of uncertainty coupled with the complex range of different judgements involved, emotions are vital in order that action can take place. But, as argued by Nussbaum (2001: 23) among others, 'we need to substitute a broader, more capricious account of cognition for the original Stoic emphasis on the grasp of linguistically formulable propositions' in order to be able to grasp that when we refer to affective bases of trust, we are not leaving a 'sociology of knowledge' perspective behind. Instead, we are merely extending and refining our understanding of *knowing* within social contexts and applying this to analyses of trust.

One further format by which past experiences, through knowledge, are drawn upon and applied in order to act amidst the present (in expectation of the future) can be conceptualised through *habitus*. As with emotion, *habitus* exists and is enacted in a less-than-conscious manner, but has been depicted here as a mechanism for approaching the future in the light of previous subjective experiences. The inculcation of particular dispositions for considering self, others and institutions in a particular light can be seen as a shorthand for ways in which tendencies towards action and decision-making are bound up with more or less conscious forms of memory, emotion, cognition and the embodied social experience (partially drawing on Young et al, 2003).

That trust is so fundamental for social life (Luhmann, 1979), and yet potentially so compromised by continued inculcating experiences within certain fields, can be seen to be reflected in the mental health of individuals. For if trust is an 'inoculation against anxiety' (Elliott, 2004), then the ways in which social experiences elicit dispositions that undermine vital 'bracketing-off' processes have significant bearings on the mental and physical day-to-day experiences of social actors. In this light, we can see that dispositions that are deemed irrational or paranoid may alternatively be considered as reflections of problematic experiences in prior social fields. The more these socio-biographical contexts are considered, the more reasonable and, indeed, rational certain decisions to trust/distrust will appear.

Notes

[1] The concept of expectations, though increasingly well developed within the Science and Technology Studies literature (for some useful work in this area, see Brown and Webster, 2004), is arguably a problematic concept within medical sociology. Researchers in this latter field tend to neglect the precise format of patients' expectations, focusing instead on problems that they *hope* (in a loose sense) clinicians can manage and/or fix.

[2] One of the underlying frameworks that informs a large body of work within psychology and economics, especially behavioural economics, is the distinction between (a) a slow, thoughtful basis of decision-making that is reflective and well-informed, and (b) a more impulsive, 'fast' approach that is based on emotions and/or basic heuristics, and which

is therefore devoid of the considered (i.e. 'rational') reflection of (a) (for an accessible introduction and synthesis of a range of studies that adopt this type of position, see Thaler and Sunstein, 2008).

[3] In this sense, we refer to a more qualified form of trust, which Calnan and Rowe (2008) distinguish from 'blind trust'. The latter could, in some ways, be considered close to Luhmann's (1979) notion of confidence, where the possibility of being let down is not even considered.

[4] We address these complex considerations in Chapter Four.

[5] Emotion and affect are used in this chapter interchangeably. In this particular sentence 'emotions' refer to the general phenomena of emotions, with 'affective experiences' referring to specific situations where emotions are 'felt' by an individual – though this experience or feeling may be conscious and/or less-than-conscious.

[6] As also included in the notes to a preceding chapter, a 'paranoid' diagnosis may often refer to the presence of positive (rather than negative) symptoms; though, in this context, it also referred to what psychiatrists interpreted as paranoid, conspiratorial delusions.

FOUR

Vulnerability and the 'will to trust'

Dependence, choice and trust

A number of questions have appeared, more or less explicitly, within the preceding chapters pertaining to a tension between processes of trust formation and the extent of choice involved within these. One example of this was in Chapter Three where we followed Barbalet in noting a 'forced option' (Barbalet, 2009: 372) aspect to trust, as was made evident in comments by participants such as 'You have to [trust] in some ways'. In Chapter One, we suggested that some degree of choice was intrinsic to trust (following Luhmann, 1988) and that this, therefore, presents us with an apparent contradiction. A number of questions thus emerge as to how we deal with the limited agency involved in trust and, where this is apparent, whether we are being accurate in referring to trust.

These concerns are latent within a number of empirical studies into the nature of trust, not least within healthcare contexts, though few studies have set out to grapple with these difficult issues. One noteworthy exception to this is a paper by Meyer and Ward (2009), which renders explicit a number of the tensions touched upon here. At the centre of these authors' concerns, and seemingly of this issue, is the notion of dependence.[1] High levels of dependence limit choice and, thus, make trust less relevant, leading Meyer and Ward to argue for a clearer distinction between when researchers are referring to trust and when – in the absence of choice – they are referring in fact to dependence.

While this would seem *prima facie* a very suitable, Luhmannian answer to this conceptual problem, there are many aspects of trust that we have visited in the previous chapters that suggest things are not quite so straightforward. The first concern with this solution is that dependence, far from being separate from trust, is in many senses a pre-condition of trust as a result of vulnerability. As was also established in Chapter One, actors only need to trust when they are vulnerable. This position of vulnerability makes salient certain power dimensions that render the vulnerable more or less inevitably dependent on certain other actors. For example, the social experience of illness within modern societies means that those experiencing morbidity are normatively oriented towards depending on those apparently able to understand, diagnose and alleviate illness – typically, healthcare experts. In trying to be more specific about when we can appropriately refer to trust, a perspective that holds trust and dependence as mutually exclusive thus hits a problem whereby the positions of vulnerability that would necessitate trust are also deemed to exclude it.

A more accurate understanding of the relationship between trust and dependence is to portray them as existing alongside one another as they are both interwoven with vulnerability; hence, one means of coping with vulnerability amidst uncertainty is through trust, but we remember that this vulnerability is also likely to render the truster dependent to a certain degree. We can deal with the linkages between dependency and trust in a more nuanced way by reflecting on the *temporality* of dependency (as touched on in Chapter One). Barbalet (2009: 382) emphasises how dependency emerges in the specific time between the giving of one's trust to a trustee and the outcome that the truster is expecting. Yet there is another aspect of dependency that is also relevant here, but which is temporally and conceptually distinct. In seeking to bring about an outcome that is 'otherwise unavailable' (Barbalet, 2009), the truster may in certain senses be reliant on certain people before there is a specific choice to trust in them. The greater the extent to which a single person or body of people monopolises the means to bring this otherwise unavailable option about (eg psychiatrists), the less choice an individual has over whether they trust or not.

Following this discussion, we can refine our understandings of these two forms of dependence in terms of chronology, agency and causality with regard to trust.

1. The form of dependency (or reliance[1]) that exists prior to trust is manifest in the *need* for the otherwise unavailable outcome, with this need seen as a feature of vulnerability (eg illness). This position limits the vulnerable person's options over whether to trust or not. This form of dependency can be seen as leading people towards processes of trust.
2. The form of dependency that exists once people have decided to trust is a feature of their decision to trust. In this sense, while the individual has a limited amount of agency (ie choice) as to whether to enter into this second format of dependency by deciding to trust (or not), once trust has been invested, there may be little remaining control (eg where one trusts a professional through disclosing sensitive information). This form of dependency thus occurs as a result of trust.

This distinction is significant in terms of analytical accuracy but, moreover, as it makes more vivid how limited agency/choice in the initial phase of dependency creates a path trajectory that may often lead to limited agency as the actor comes to place their trust. These issues of time become more complicated, though, when we consider the nature of mental illness and its chronicity. Where healthcare relationships are ongoing (see Thorne and Robinson, 1989), trust is accordingly negotiated over time and best described as a process (eg Khodyakov, 2007) rather than being reducible to a one-off decision.[2]

This clarification of the nature of dependency and trust in the midst of vulnerability forms the foundations upon which the analysis presented in the remainder of this chapter is built. Developing understandings of the ways in which tendencies towards trust are embedded within structures of vulnerability will be the central aim of this chapter, alongside working through some of the paradoxes between choice and dependency that have been raised thus far. Crucial to the development of the chapter is a further tension that exists between the precision required for accurate theoretical considerations of trust on the one hand, and the much more 'messy' empirical realities of trust within everyday settings on the other. By working within this tension, it is hoped that our data will aid the refinement of theory while an enhanced conceptual apparatus will enhance our understandings of trust in empirical settings. With these ends in mind, we begin in the next section by rehearsing some of the very specific distinctions developed by Luhmann (1979, 1988) before moving into more empirical settings and exploring the utility of Luhmannian insights when considering the types of choices actors make within trust processes. We then consider the extent to which trust and mistrust may exist concomitantly within empirical settings before returning to more theoretical avenues in terms of actors' 'will to trust' (Brown, 2009a), the relevance of 'leaps of faith' (Möllering, 2001) and hope, and the salience of *habitus* for understanding how people trust when exceedingly vulnerable (Pilgrim et al, 2011).

Luhmannian insights: choice, regret and attribution

The two relatively short works on trust by Niklas Luhmann (1979, 1988) are highly influential within the trust literature and have featured prominently within more recent sociological accounts of trust (Möllering, 2001).[3] One great strength of these two studies, as we have noted, is Luhmann's readiness to distinguish trust from what it is not – for example, confidence and familiarity (see Chapter One). Fundamental to the distinguishing marks of trust is reflexivity (Calnan and Rowe, 2008; Meyer and Ward, 2009), or rather a number of reflexivities:

1. Trust is different from confidence in that the former process involves acting while being aware of the possibility of negative outcomes occurring – of being let down.
2. Moreover, 'trust is only required if a bad outcome would make you regret your action' (Luhmann, 1988: 98). In this sense, we cannot say one trusts by following a particular route when the alternative is worse – for example, likely death. Hence, a notion of reflexivity around alternatives becomes apparent.
3. Following on from point 2, we can see that trust differs from familiarity in that it involves a particular setting, where apparent 'risk' is confronted, and where a choice must be made. It is in the midst of this choice that, for Luhmann, trust becomes relevant.

The issue of being aware of the possibility of negative outcomes is comparatively straightforward in terms of the considerations we are addressing here. However, the need for a genuine dilemma over options, where the potential for regret exists along either option, suggests that we should be very careful when referring to trust in healthcare contexts. Following this line of argument, we might argue that an individual diagnosed with cancer has no option but to receive treatment, and, therefore, that trust is irrelevant. Or, even where an alternative is perceived to exist by the actor, such as complementary medicine, this would need to be a distinctly credible and mutually exclusive alternative for the concept of trust to be appropriately invoked by social scientists trying to understand this context. The issue of *regret* will be returned to in the next section.

Associated with the reflexivity and regret in relation to choice, Luhmann also raises the important notion of attribution when referring to the distinctness of trust (Meyer and Ward, 2009). Rooted in the reflexivity that is central to choice, a bad decision is regretted in a sense that the blame for the failure or bad outcome is oriented by the truster towards him- or herself. It was a poor selection on the part of the truster which led to the negative consequences that are later experienced (Meyer and Ward, 2009). In contrast, when people are in a state of confidence – in that they are unaware of the potential negative outcome –they attribute the failures externally: the supposedly reliable individual or institution is at fault for dysfunction, rather than the individual who had held them in confident regard (Luhmann, 1988; Meyer and Ward, 2009).

Yet, as the overly neat format of this last distinction indicates, it can be considered appropriate to theorise or research trust from a Luhmannian position while not assuming that the behaviours he considers – through notions of trust, confidence and familiarity – are as clearly delineated as he depicts. It is easy to think of examples from an array of settings, not least our research amidst psychosis services, where the regret and blame after being let down are attributed both internally and externally – a frustration with oneself for trusting coupled to a resentment or anger towards a particular professional for failing to provide a good-quality outcome. Luhmann's working distinctions are, therefore, perhaps best viewed as highly sophisticated ideal-types – very helpful for us in orienting the analysis of real social contexts, and yet we should not necessarily expect to find empirical contexts amenable to such neat categorisations.

Second, we might take issue with Luhmann's consideration of the basic purpose of trust – in fending against complexity. As with uncertainty, complexity is not necessarily problematic and, indeed, recent health policies in the UK have sought to *create* choice, rather than overcome the problems of choice. Rather, complexity becomes a problem when the uncertainty associated with it exists concomitantly with vulnerability, and where these joint conditions give rise to anxiety. By seeing trust as a solution to anxiety (Elliott, 2004) rather than complexity per se, our focus on the types of choices we make when in conditions associated with trust come to be seen somewhat differently. Again, this thread will be developed further in the next section.

Finally, in the light of our discussions in Chapter Three, we can also develop a positive critique of Luhmannian notions of trust in terms of the nature and time frame of the decisions involved. We argued in the preceding chapter that the formats by which knowledge is applied within contexts of uncertainty and vulnerability (or complexity) are, in many senses, affective and embodied, as well as pertaining to notions of social space. We also suggested, via considerations of *habitus* (Misztal, 1996), that we ought to reconsider the chronology across which knowledge is applied. Whereas Luhmann refers to very distinct time frames and specific decisional contexts, it may be useful to maintain the idea of a specific context in which trust is relevant while also being aware that knowledge may be applied as part of a longer-running process of trust – rather than focusing too narrowly upon distinct decisions.

Choosing or not choosing? Recognising agency amidst structures

In many healthcare settings, it can be argued that choices of whether to accept certain types of treatment are limited. As referred to by many of the coronary heart disease patients interviewed in Meyer and Ward's (2009) study, they had little option other than to comply with the biomedical hegemony as embodied by the particular professionals treating them. In this sense, they were depending or relying on these professionals rather than choosing between alternative options. This echoes our own recent research into trust relations where individuals with cervical cancer (Brown, 2009a), diabetes or who were in need of hip surgery (Calnan and Rowe, 2008: 163)[4] generally perceived medical treatment through the NHS as the only viable route.

In some senses, the service users we interviewed in this current research had somewhat different experiences. Many referred to their first experiences with mental health services as episodes when they were ill but where they did not see themselves as ill at the time. In this sense, there were a number of alternative routes for them to follow other than mental health services and the option was clearly there for them to trust or not. In some of these accounts, however, mental healthcare was imposed upon service users, either through involuntary treatment, through demands placed on them regarding whether they were still able to look after their children or where they described themselves as being so ill that they were not able to object to treatment. For these latter service users, choice was annihilated by their illness contexts.

Over the longer term, however, it would seem that many more options were open to these service users. Only one of the service users was under the care of an assertive outreach team where he had no option at all but to cooperate with a treatment plan. *Prima facie*, the other respondents were all sufficiently at liberty, and sufficiently well, to choose their level of cooperation with services in the community. However, all eight referred to their options being limited in some manner, at least to some degree. Largely, this seemed due to their experience of vulnerability, their associated need for help and their perception of mental health services as the main viable alternative.

Of the eight service users we interviewed, the least embedded within norms of care was arguably a young man without a diagnosis. He had experienced two 'breakdowns', and had been referred to an Early Intervention in Psychosis service by his family doctor. He did not perceive his vulnerability as psychosis–related, but, nonetheless, wanted help to cope better with things:

> "And the 'Early Interventions' discharged me … around September [year] and said 'If there's ever a problem again come back to us'. I came back to them, I don't know why, all I know is if there's something that can be done, it has to be done, so then I'm back with Early Interventions with a different woman from the autumn." (*Service user 6*)

Here, in spite of no specific illness, and no certainty that the service could help, the choice exercised by this participant to be involved with services is very much embedded within his need for help and his perception of the service as the only viable alternative:

> "They said, 'Look, your GP has said that you've said some fairly worrying things and your GP has said we're probably the best people to help', at which stage I started seeing the 'Early Interventions'. They put me down a route which probably wasn't right for me and that route has kind of been and gone, and yet the 'Early Interventions' are kind of the people who know me and the 'Early Interventions' are sort of looking at other things I could do, which isn't actually Early Intervention." (*Service user 6*)

In this case, the awareness of his need and vulnerability, the way in which there was an existing relationship with the service, and that the service represented a more or less direct route to help seemed to compel this man to cooperation. As he noted in the first excerpt, it "has to be done".

So, although *prima facie* this service user had a range of options open to him and no apparent compulsion, his needs and lack of clear alternatives to meet these needs rendered his decisions highly bounded – with perceived choice accordingly limited. Choice was even more curtailed (or decimated in some cases) within the accounts of service users when referring to their experiences as involuntary inpatients. The following service user, the one still in contact with the assertive outreach team, described his alternatives around medication during a phase as an inpatient accordingly:

> "Yeah. Not that I had any choice in it because of course as I say, you know … when I said to a nurse, 'What happens if I don't take the pills?', they said, 'Well yeah but you'll never ever get out of hospital in your life'. You know?" (*Service user 1*)

Yet, despite these more or less obvious limitations to choice, it would be incorrect to describe these two service users (and others) as utterly lacking choice. Nor, in reference to Luhmann, would it be appropriate to argue that they did not run the risk of regret and that this regret would be internally attributed.

As implied earlier, and made clear in these two contrasting positions, we may usefully and accurately refer to choice as being more or less embedded within contexts that are social in nature, rather than seeing choice as a simple dichotomy – choice or no choice. That service user 6 (quoted earlier) was discharged, and remained so for a number of months, before re-approaching the Early Intervention Service, suggests an element of choice remained. However, we can say that the alternative between being in contact with the service and remaining outside of assistance was embedded within notions of hope, or a 'will to trust' (Brown, 2009a), by which his vulnerability and need for a solution led him to feel compelled to continue working with the Early Intervention team. As a result of this embedded choice (as opposed to totally unconstrained choice), his hope in some format of a solution (which enables and compels his trust) means that he leaves himself open to regret; potentially, he may see himself as being let down in the future.

The experiences as described by service user 1 (also quoted earlier) can, to some degree, be analysed differently. His legal and medical status as an involuntary patient meant he had no choice as to whether to receive particular medication treatment (eg 'depo' injections) or not. However, this lack of choice over this significant aspect of his treatment is not to say choice was totally absent in this situation. Nor would it be correct for us to say that his agency was utterly limited even with regards to the forcibly administered medication. As well as acting to choose whether or not to follow a certain path, we can describe patients or service users as choosing and continuing to act in terms of how they respond once along a certain path. Examples of this action include accepting this path positively and developing positive expectations as this path is ventured along (trust), or whether this path is perceived negatively, as likely to fail, and as provoking anxiety (mistrust). Accounts of inpatient experiences, though typified by a lack of choice in a number of senses, nonetheless display choice over this form of reaction (relative acceptance or anxiety) and a related format of expectation (more positive or negative).

These different types of reaction can, therefore, be seen as behaviours, highlighting agency in spite of an apparent lack of choice. Furthermore, the more positive or negative reactions and expectations continue to fulfil Luhmann's criteria of 'regret' – with those with more positive expectations arguably liable to greater feelings of being let down and notions of blaming oneself for continuing to expect positive outcomes. In this sense, we see that trust is relevant in describing far more than what occurs in the relatively brief temporal moment of the 'crossroads'. If, instead, we recognise trust as an ongoing process of intra- and interpersonal negotiation, we can see relationships within healthcare contexts as *continually* involving choice, action, dependence *and* more positive or negative formats of expectations.

These ongoing negotiations of trust were apparent right across our respondents, even within the contexts of involuntary inpatient experiences (see also Riordan and Humphreys, 2007). In the following excerpt, a service user refers to the lack of choice in certain aspects of his experience, but he also describes how he continued to exercise control and choice over how much he disclosed to people about his concerns. In this manner, trust is very relevant:

> "I think if someone spent time to get to know me and that it's not just about the daily routine, you know, where you've got to take medication and you've got to go to mealtimes and you've got to keep your room tidy, you've got to have a wash or a shave or whatever, which is daily routine stuff, anyone can do that. But if they've obviously sat down next to me and had a chat and tried to get to know me a little bit, I feel that I would probably go to them for help." (*Service user 7*)

Here, in spite of the manifold limitations of choice in healthcare and, indeed, over so many aspects of his daily life, he continues to exercise control, choice and trust in his disclosure (or lack thereof) with certain professionals on the inpatient ward.

The messiness of real world trust: trust and mistrust alongside one another

As argued in the previous section, we should still hold trust as highly relevant in understanding the experiences of service users and patients even when their choice over treatment is apparently limited. In trust research within the context of gynaecological cancer, where almost no alternative other than to pursue treatment was perceived, patients referred to a range of more or less trusting perspectives – both towards the professionals who were treating them and their healthcare contexts more broadly (Brown, 2009a). Some of these patients referred to high levels of trust and experienced comparatively limited anxiety, while others said that they did not trust and suffered comparatively significant anxiety and concern. In both contexts of mental illness and gynaecological cancer, choice over treatment options are intertwined with, but not the same as, choice as to whether to trust or not.

As we delve deeper into the accounts of patients or service users, and acknowledge the multiple forms of choice, dependency and agency, not to mention the varying degrees to which choice and agency are embedded within broader contexts, the whole picture of trust emerges as an increasingly complex one. Our framework for considering trust becomes still further convoluted when we note examples of where trust and mistrust exist concomitantly. From a purely theoretical perspective, such a phenomenon should not occur; either people trust in their healthcare via a particular professional, or they do not (distrust) or they actively mistrust. Yet such is the multidimensionality of healthcare – as regards expertise, institutions, different professionals and so on– and such is the nuanced way in which these different aspects of trust interact to enable expectations (see Chapter Two), that it is possible that positive expectations exist in spite of the truster being decidedly mindful of the profoundly negative expectations that would appear to contradict these.

Brown and colleagues (2011b: 285) refer to findings from interviews with gynae-oncology patients, noting that 'the sample included women who reported very high levels of trust, distinctly problematic mistrust, and the more common scenarios by which levels of trust and a poignant awareness of the limitations of trust (and thus anxiety) existed concomitantly'. These combined experiences of trust and anxiety can in some ways be viewed as a feature of what is at stake in the midst of cancer. It is perhaps unsurprising that trust did not enable these women to totally overcome their concerns, and that grave fears about the future continued to linger or remained starkly prominent. Yet other studies, including those into healthcare contexts with arguably less extreme emotional experiences than cancer, also note the existence of trust alongside mistrust. For example, Haddow and Cunningham-Burley (2008) describe accounts of public perceptions of a genetic database and draw attention to the number of sources of knowledge that trusters drew upon, the relative strengths and impacts of these within their consciousness, and the complexities and futuristic projections that had to be accounted for. These features underlined the *messiness* of trust within this study – and, at the same time, its teleology in the way that levels of trust facilitated action even in the parallel presence of mistrust.

Similar experiences of trust existing alongside mistrust were apparent within our data – in the accounts of service users and professionals. Here, one manager refers to the difficulty in trusting service users and how the trust that facilitates relationships exists alongside a more cynical, mistrustful awareness of the dark side of trust:

> "Well, you can trust implicitly without actually being mindful of [it] … I think it's a danger that you have to guard against....
>
> You're actually not doing your job. I mean there are times when I have to sort of question … you know, I've been speaking to this particular patient, [thinking]: 'Why are they saying this?' 'Have you been…?' 'Have you done this?' 'Have you done that?' If they're actually saying to me, 'Yes and this is my rationale', and what have you, I will then say, 'Right, well OK, you need to record that so that it's there'. And I have to trust what they actually are telling me." (*Manager*)

This account brings to light a number of the tensions apparent with trust decisions amidst uncertainty and the way choices are embedded within particular contexts. From one perspective, a professional's need to develop a relationship with a particular service user constrains choice – meaning that the professional has little option but to trust. Yet once this path has been ventured along, the reaction of the professional means that amidst this trust, there exists another sense of mistrust, or distrust, rooted in past experiences of trusting service users and occasions where this trust has been disappointed – with serious consequences. These two considerations, existing somewhat uneasily alongside one another, are a product of the multiple dimensions and sources of knowledge that are drawn upon when trusting and the way these must be applied within certain social contexts – for example, when a service user comes across in a compelling manner but their notes refer to a personality disorder. A further tension is visible in terms of the 'implicit' trust that is also referred to by the manager, suggesting different degrees of consciousness when trust 'decisions' are taken. Here, we might argue that two different forms of *habitus*, the personal (trusting) and the professional (wariness of trusting), are brought together, resulting in the more or less conscious tensions between the two.

The extent to which choice is able to be exercised has been seen here as an important feature in the way trust or mistrust may work alongside one another. As discussed earlier, choice is far from a simple binary and, therefore, cannot be used as a straightforward basis for distinguishing trust from other separate concepts of processes (c.f. Luhmann, 1988). Yet it would be a mistake to discount notions of choice as irrelevant to our understanding. Indeed, the nature of choice, and the extent to which choice is bounded by the social environment – embedded within particular contextual norms – adds much to our analysis of the complex experiences of trust within empirical contexts.

Vulnerability and a 'will to trust'

This boundedness of choice, which is salient for trust, has been seen in earlier sections of this chapter to be very much socially constructed. Whether this boundedness is rooted in norms of professional obligation, the hegemonic position of biomedical approaches to cancer or the hope of some as-yet-unknown solution to a position of vulnerability, it is often the lifeworld of an individual or institution that limits choices related to trust. The latter notion referred to here, that of *hope*, would seem to be another concept that aids us in our understanding of trust.

Previous studies have noted the existence of a willingness or will to trust (eg Lee-Treweek, 2002; Möllering, 2006), which is decisive in leading to the 'leap of faith' that is always necessary for trust to overcome uncertainty (Möllering, 2001). Vulnerability has been seen as relevant in fuelling this will to trust (see Chapter Three; also Brown, 2009a). Indeed, heightened levels of vulnerability have been associated with a stronger will to trust, where this has been understood as rational due to the greater utility of trust in this context (Brown, 2009a, 2011). So, in looking to the social context from which trust emerges as a way of understanding how choice may be constrained, it would seem that the level of vulnerability experienced within such a context will shape the nature and extent of an actor's 'choice' to trust. This framework may be useful in developing understandings of the different phases of trust across the timeline of chronic illness experience (see Box 4.1).

Box 4.1: Changing trust dynamics over time

Thorne and Robinson's (1989) study of patients with chronic illness distinguished between the 'naive trust' typical of the start of clinician–patient relations and 'reconstructed trust', trust that was re-established by patients after experiencing a period of disenchantment with their provider. The extent and way in which trust was reconstructed affected the type of clinician–patient relationship, varying from 'hero worship' when trust was re-established by designating an individual healthcare professional distinct from all others, to trust, to 'resignation' when there was little evidence of any trust.

Certainly, the accounts of service users interviewed for our study suggested a variation of experiences and levels of trust across the period of chronic illness management recounted within interviews. However, in contrast to the findings of Thorne and Robinson, initial attitudes towards services and individual professionals were typically closer to forms of wariness and scepticism, rather than 'naive trust':

"I didn't really understand what was going wrong with me, I was quite confused I suppose, cos they [professionals] were trying to explain to me that there is a mental health issue here, and I'm believing that there isn't, you know – if anything it was all positive for me, it was all a good thing. But that's the hyper-manic….

So it took a few weeks to get them to understand what really is going on, and for me to understand that there is stuff going on." (Julie)

Often, however, service users were able to form trusting relationships and these typically were described in terms of certain significant characteristics of professionals (though 'hero worship' would be an exaggeration in most cases), which enabled them to trust after previous misgivings. Both service user and professional accounts referred to the divulging of weakness on the part of the professional (within certain limits of appropriateness) as an important basis of trust. As one professional noted – 'showing that you're human' – or as this service user describes:

"She [support worker] is one that has gone through an experience [of mental health problems] herself so I find it really easy to talk to her, I ask her advice and stuff and she gives me really good advice, you know." (Julie)

The way choices regarding trust are embedded within vulnerability should not, as underlined earlier, be mistaken for a lack of agency on the part of the truster. Indeed, empirical analysis of the will to trust points to the highly 'active role of the truster' in 'bracketing off' aspects of uncertainty or possibilities of negative outcomes – as a means of focusing upon and, in some senses, creating positive expectations (Brown, 2009a). This emphasis upon the creative role of the truster in managing their 'subjective gaze' (Brown, 2009a) adds a further nuance to our understandings of the way constrained choice shapes trust, rather than ruling it out as irrelevant. The tensions that exist within this subjectivity (Kierkegaard, 1957), mirroring some of the apparent contradictions referred to in the previous section, require further theorising. In the pursuit of this end, notions of emotion work (Hochschild, 1979) and 'aintegration' (Lomranz and Benyamini, 2009) represent potentially fruitful pathways.

Yet, while there exist more conscious paths by which trust may be fashioned in the midst of vulnerability, research also points towards other less-than-conscious routes. One interest that has emerged within our previous research is the different formats and tendencies of trust formation within different domains of medicine (eg Calnan and Rowe, 2008). For example, there is a stark contrast between the way trust is won within the acute experience of an Accident and Emergency (A&E) department and the way trust must be qualified within more chronic care contexts (Dibben and Lean, 2003). This difference is summed up neatly by this A&E Registrar from a previous study (Brown, 2008c: 194–5):

> *A&E Registrar:* "In emergency care you're very vulnerable, in some ways it's nice for me, but they're very, very vulnerable hence they trust you."

> *Interviewer:* "Because they have to?"

> *A&E Registrar:* "Because they have to. And I've done that before when I've injured myself. You just put yourself in … [their hands] … you know."

Hence, there is something about the nature of vulnerability that greatly facilitates trust within this type of setting. That is not to say that any person in an acute context, such as A&E, will trust; but, rather, that acute vulnerability makes trust easier to accomplish.

Pilgrim and colleagues (2011) develop a useful understanding of this link between heightened levels of vulnerability and trust by returning to notions of dependence. The framework they consider can be seen as highly congruent with the ideas around trust and *habitus* developed in the previous chapter. The socio-biography of an individual, where early childhood is especially significant, shapes certain dispositions as to the extent to which one tends to rely on others and, indeed, oneself. The authors argue that 'the developmental challenge to balance interdependency and personal autonomy is thus thrown into relief during times of illness and healthcare utilization' (Pilgrim et al, 2011: 44), where more basic dispositions thus become apparent – such as dependence or resentment:

> During times of acute sickness dependency can be evident in both an objective and subjective sense. On the first count we really might need others to tend to our basic needs of feeding and toileting in the manner of an infant. On the second count feeling ill brings with it

regressive feelings of anxiety, pain and the need for comfort. (Pilgrim et al, 2011: 44)

The latter sentence of this quotation points to the salient role of emotions within this *habitus*, whereby experiences of certain types of sensations and vulnerabilities, and affective reactions to these, led the actor to adopt a certain type of response. *Habitus* and emotions thus render this response grounded in socio-biographies. Past experiences of others as sources of help and support, or as figures of neglect and abuse, will inculcate dispositions that become especially prominent in times of extreme vulnerability (Pilgrim et al, 2011).

The more chronic experience of vulnerability amidst mental illness suggests a quite different format of dependence and trust than the acute example of A&E care noted earlier. Yet most of our service user respondents referred to oscillating phases between relative health and illness, and associated levels of vulnerability. Occasionally, severe lapses into more serious experiences of illness were, in many senses, 'acute' episodes. But, in either shorter- or longer-term formats, the responses amidst vulnerability can be seen as being influenced by emotional responses within this vulnerability and through other dispositions shaped by a range of social fields encountered over the life-course. In being shaped by and thus oriented towards certain enduring social contexts, these dispositions are in themselves 'ecologically rational', oriented as they are towards unfamiliar situations (Gigerenzer and Brighton, 2009).

Disproportionately frequent experiences of being let down when vulnerable, which are associated with the aetiology of poor mental health, may also compromise service users' dispositions towards trust (Pilgrim et al, 2011), as *habitus*-shaping experiences. This can be seen as a serious challenge to services, as noted by many of the professionals we interviewed. These dispositions were less clearly evident within service user accounts; though this is likely to be partly an artefact of the less-than-conscious status of *habitus*, and especially the self-selecting aspects of recruitment by which the least trusting were also less likely to participate in our research. Yet, even where trust was reported by service users as highly limited, cooperation around treatment was still possible; though, again, we see the role of creative agency on the part of the service user as vital to this (see Box 2.2).

Conclusion

The background to this chapter is the tension that exists within various aspects of the trust literature regarding associations between trust and choice – as prompted by Luhmann (1979) and as recently rendered explicit by Meyer and Ward (2009). Following Luhmann's (1979, 1988) highly relevant concerns that the concept of trust is applied too loosely (thus losing analytical effectiveness and accuracy), there has been a concern to distinguish trust from other concepts on the basis of choice (among other considerations). This poses the problem of how considerations of vulnerability, which makes trust necessary while greatly impinging upon choice, should be related to trust. In grappling with these concerns, which are highly salient to analyses of trust (especially within healthcare contexts), we have developed a number of arguments that contribute to understandings within this debate. Far from solving these conundrums, and perhaps acting to further complicate in some instances, the goal of this chapter has been to extend and refine analyses of trust within situations of vulnerability.

Central to the framework developed in these sections has been a more nuanced consideration of choice that overcomes the limitations of a simplistic choice–no-choice dualism. By seeing choice as bounded by, and embedded within, a range of contextual factors – of which vulnerability is key – we are able to accommodate understandings of limited choice and the way this impacts on trust, rather than insisting that anything other than totally unconstrained choice renders trust irrelevant.

Furthermore, the significance of different time dimensions within choice, and, indeed, within dependence as a result of certain choices (or limitations of choice), has also been seen to be highly relevant to analyses – offering a more detailed understanding of the ways in which choice, dependence and trust impact on one another within social processes. Understanding trust as a process (Khodyakov, 2007), rather than a one-off decision, is accordingly significant in incorporating and describing the agency of trusters – even amidst conditions of dependence – as well as offering a more accurate conception of trust within dynamic social relations. Trust is decisive to understanding certain 'decision moments' that invariably are vital to healthcare outcomes, yet the expectations that are central to trust are not momentary phenomena in themselves. This ongoing process of trust and its dynamic development within certain relationships is especially apparent within the chronic treatment contexts of mental health services.

All of these aspects are relevant in considering the 'will to trust', which enables the 'leap of faith' that is necessary for trust (Möllering, 2006), in order to overcome the unknowables that characterise situations where trust is relevant. In describing factors that orient and drive this willingness (or reluctance as the case may be), notions of vulnerability, hope and *habitus* have been seen as significant in understanding the social forces that bear upon actors:

- Actors' agency in decisions to trust (or not) is certainly embedded within their positions of vulnerability and associated power dynamics. This existing position (in its relation to power) is likely to influence the range of available options perceived by the actor. Such 'choice' is also very much embedded within actors' past experiences of the *competence* of experts/colleagues/institutions/ service users, as well as the extent to which they have found that the *motives* of similar experts/colleagues/institutions/service users in the past have been congruent with their own interests. Furthermore, vulnerability shapes the level of utility trust can provide, in terms of the experienced 'need' for help in managing vulnerability and the associated value attached to attaining a particular (otherwise unavailable) end.

- Hope is bound up with these latter aspects. Certain socially structured contexts may inculcate an individual with a *habitus* towards generally positive expectations about the likelihood of quality outcomes. This generalised hope in the potential for positive futures facilitates a strong will to trust, as do highly vulnerable situations in that hope is in some senses forged within situations of despair (Schrank et al, 2008; Brown, 2011) and the need to cope with and overcome such problematic contexts.

- As the preceding points indicate, rather than seeing hopefulness as some 'innate' character trait, we can instead conceptualise a range of general tendencies that facilitate or inhibit trust and analyse these as dispositions inculcated by specific socio-biographic contexts – as characterised by immediate vulnerabilities and related needs to cope, as well as a deeper set of dispositions inculcated over the life-course. Thus, past and more immediate experiences within certain fields are significant (often less than consciously) in shaping dispositions towards others, towards the self and towards trust.

Notes

[1] What we refer to here as dependence might also be referred to as reliance, depending on the active or passive position of patients or service users. Where patients or service users are more active – for example, in certain cases of expert patients and their management of diabetes –reliance might be more appropriate than dependence. We refer further to differences between chronic and acute care, and levels of dependence, later in this chapter.

[2] Though, as we argued in Chapter One, even in non-chronic contexts, trust is best seen as a relational process rather than reduced to notions of a one-off decision.

[3] For a useful genealogy of sociologies of trust, see Möllering (2001).

[4] In Calnan and Rowe's (2008) study, patients reported that they were rarely actively involved in decisions about where to be referred – with performance data only being drawn upon to check out the doctor or organisation after a referral decision was made:

> "What choice does a layman have? To have choice, to exercise choice, you need knowledge and we do not have that so when I was told who the surgeon would be, whose team I was going to be referred to I then started searching on the Internet. There is a web site that gives you the star ratings of the various hospitals. Dr A came up very well and after talking to friends it appears that by chance I have landed at the door of the top hip man so I was very happy about that and fortunate." (Hip patient 11, quoted in Calnan and Rowe, 2008: 163).

FIVE

The difficulties of *trust-work* within a paradigm of risk

Thus far, much attention has been paid to the contexts of vulnerability and uncertainty that make trust relevant and salient for service users. We have briefly noted in earlier chapters that mental health professionals deal with manifold uncertainties, though the ways in which these uncertainties are intertwined with high levels of vulnerability have not been discussed in any significant depth up to this point. This chapter begins by noting how professionals respond to vulnerability and how these responses are shaped by institutional and policy contexts. We assess the format of risk approaches that aims at control and explore the 'trust–control dialectic' (Gallivan and Depledge, 2003; Brown, 2008a) that results within mental health contexts. This provides one useful basis for considering the interrelatedness of different levels of trust: manager–professional, inter-professional and professional–service user. Drawing on our data, we go on to consider the appearance of virtuous or vicious circles of trust, and the way these cyclical patterns are rooted in institutional policy formats on the one hand, and the social contexts of service users on the other. The chapter will close with some initial policy recommendations, drawing on some of the notions of transaction cost economics touched upon in earlier chapters, which will lay the basis for certain discussions that will be pursued in the final chapter of this book.

Professionals in the midst of vulnerability

The preceding chapter explored various features of the responses of service users, in many cases leaning towards trust, which were understood within social contexts of vulnerability and the needs of service users to cope with this. Mental health service users, especially those with diagnoses of psychosis, are often characterised as a vulnerable group, but less attention is paid to the vulnerability experienced by professionals. Earlier chapters referred to the close linkages between risk and blame (following Douglas, 1992) and, moreover, the way risk has become a defining concept of recent mental health policy in England (Pilgrim, 2007). In contrast to neighbouring policy contexts, Scotland being one notable example (Darjee and Crichton, 2004), significant emphasis has been especially placed upon certain forms of risk management within English mental health services (Langan, 2010).

The very nature of risk, especially in terms of its application within modern organisation contexts, is to apportion blame (Douglas, 1992), often onto the shoulders of experts (Luhmann, 1993). Risk was a significant theme in professionals' accounts of their day-to-day work. Concerns regarding blame, and associated experiences of vulnerability, were similarly prominent. The following excerpt is quoted at length as it draws out a number of such aspects of the vulnerability faced by professionals:

> *Interviewer:* "Would you say you or your colleagues feel vulnerable to having made bad [decisions] … or decisions which later turned out to be wrong …?"

> *Psychologist:* "Yes. I think we do because a bad decision can have such dreadful consequences."

> *Interviewer:* "So that would be more the consequences for the service user as opposed to the ramifications say from the [NHS] Trust …"

> *Psychologist:* "I think it probably would be more from the point of view of the service user but only just. You know, it's a very important thing for myself and for colleagues too because the consequences can be desperate for us too, yeah."

> *Interviewer:* "And so does that have an impact on how you make decisions or the outcomes of decisions, do you think?"

> *Psychologist:* "Yeah. Some of the anxiety that I'm mentioning about record-keeping is about that, it's about trying to make sure that, when you've made a decision you can't be certain about, you've put in the record as much about the process of decision-making that you possibly could."

As this psychologist suggests, and as was discussed regarding service users in Chapter One, vulnerability exists alongside uncertainty but, in many senses, is bound up with it. The unknowable outcomes that are inherent to this form of work, and the potentially 'dreadful' consequences attached to certain outcomes, renders professionals exceedingly vulnerable to guilt, blame and institutional sanctions where they are seen to be seriously at fault. Warner (2006) describes the way that risk-oriented knowledge, partially generated by high-profile inquiries into past failures, becomes ingrained within the working perspectives and attitudes of mental health services and individual professionals in particular. Accordingly, professionals become increasingly reflexive with regard to the 'conduct' of their professional conduct,[1] and as these professional-subjects are recast within particular knowledge frameworks, so a 'bureaumentality' becomes pervasive (Sterne, 2003).

This heightened reflexivity generates associated costs for the mental health of mental health professionals. These pressures and concerns around blame, exacerbated by policy and institutional responses within current policy frameworks, exist alongside the stresses and strains of working with a vulnerable – sometimes distressed and unpredictable – client group where, once again, uncertainty is a distinct and underlying phenomenon:

> "The thing that I find difficult.... Do you know what, it's just so different, every day just facing different issues on a day-to-day basis and that's really quite stressful. And it's just … you know, the whole job is … you just don't know what's going to come up with each client and I think that's the thing. Because you're learning as you go on and just knowing whether you've made the decision or not, really in terms of keeping that client safe or not, that's what is difficult I'd say. I mean obviously, you know, there are issues around paperwork and keeping up to date with that as well, that's difficult in itself; making sure everything's on the computer and you've got it all up to date, but it's just being faced with different scenarios every day and not knowing whether you've done the right thing or not by that client." (*Community Psychiatric Nurse [CPN]*)

In the midst of these characteristics and pressures of their work, professionals may react in different ways in order to manage uncertainty and vulnerability. As discussed in earlier chapters, these modes of action often tend towards one of two directions: trust and relational approaches on the one hand; or risk management and attempts at more bureaucratic forms of control on the other. The format and direction of reactions are very much embedded within the organisational and institutional contexts in which professionals work as well as power dynamics relating to the experience, seniority and profession of a particular worker.

That mental health organisations and management has moved towards a more risk-oriented and bureaucratised format ensured that this was a common mechanism for managing vulnerability. Almost all professionals referred to the paperwork element of their job and especially emphasised the defensive, 'back-covering' aspects of this mode of behaviour:

> "They [managers] want you to record every conversation, every text. Now for some of my carers and clients that can be 10, 20 a day and that's … and it probably takes about 5 or 10 minutes to put each contact on so you can imagine … that's something that … and it's not necessarily a negative because obviously we need to be recording what we do, but it's a shame that we couldn't use a bit more scope and the reason is, is because I know they're covering their backs because if a client ever said, 'I sent you that text' or 'I made that phone call', and you haven't got a record of it, then you'd be pulled up on it." (*Social worker*)

Professionals thus resort to bureaucratic modes of managing vulnerability due to the organisational-managerial pressures, expectations and blame-related conventions. The way they themselves are checked and monitored, as opposed to being simply trusted to carry out their work, has implications for how they deal with clients. Thus, in the preceding example, the defensive approach to clients, recording what they say rather than trusting clients not to complain, was a product of the broader organisational context.

Professionals, morality and the trust–control dialectic

Professionals did not solely resort to checking/control approaches to managing their vulnerability, even though the organisational context pushed them in such a direction. Also clear was a certain 'will to trust' among our professional participants[2] – as described by a number of professionals and as was referred to in the previous chapter: "I have to trust what they actually are telling me".

From a certain perspective, it might be said that there is a professional *duty* to trust. The power and authority of professionals and the vocational aspects of their work impose a moral obligation to be trustworthy, yet, as Pilgrim and colleagues argue (2011: 157), the special relationship that exists between professional and patients is, furthermore, marked by assumptions of 'mutuality', 'informality and cooperation'. Within this normative and ethical setting, there is thus a moral preference for utilising trust relations, as opposed to checking and control, which is explained by far more than simply the efficacy of the former. Trusting service users was often seen as the *appropriate* course of action towards service users – following Simmel (1950), there would seem to be 'a high moral value to trust which makes it a rather special medium of social exchange' (Möllering, 2001: 407); although, as discussed in the preceding chapter, professionals also referred to a professional responsibility that this trust should be qualified and not simply 'blind trust'.

This latter feature of 'conditional trust' (Calnan and Rowe, 2008) alludes to the tension that exists between trust-based approaches and control – a relationship that is far more complex than one simply being the alternative to the other. Indeed, Möllering (2005) emphasises the duality of trust and control, with trust only possible through its ability to enact aspects of control and control always reliant on certain aspects of trust[3] (Brown and Calnan [2011] apply this understanding within a healthcare context). Building on this notion of trust and control as a duality, or a dialectic (see Brown, 2008a; following Gallivan and Depledge, 2003), we have argued elsewhere that the application of control mechanisms may not only replace trust in the short term, but may, furthermore, undermine the possibilities for trusting behaviour in the longer term (Brown and Calnan, 2011). Control mechanisms tend to create more instrumental, goal-oriented, formats of behaviour (Brown, 2008b) and these are prone to impinging upon the communicative rationality of healthcare environments. Trust is rooted in the relational dynamics of the latter and, therefore, the colonisation of interactive lifeworlds by the bureaucratic aspects of control (Habermas, 1987) is problematic:

"And more [bureaucracy] added to it every day. And so that means that a lot of it I think is duplication. And that actually writing something down and saying this ... that should be enough, rather than actually doing it in a different format for something else and a different format for something else. It actually cuts down the face–to–face client contact." (*CPN and social worker*[4])

"... if you want to do the paperwork and see the client, then you need to reduce the visits, reduce the appointments and, you know.... So that is the thing, basically I don't like it. And like, you know, we need to do [paperwork] but, you know, sometimes it's too much." (*Social worker*)

There is a concern, therefore, that as time with clients is impinged upon, and as a 'bureaumentality' is encouraged, the quality and refinement of relationships and mutual understanding suffers (Davidsen and Reventlow, 2010), thus constraining possibilities for trust:

"You know, like a rapport then depends on the caseload and the, you know, pressure we get ... so I would say the last clients on my list may not be ... may not have that because I don't have enough time to spend with them. So obviously things, you know, external factors, affect it [the rapport] and ... the trust also." (*Social worker*)

Thus, we have a situation where control impinges upon time, communication and rapport, which are all salient to the creation of trust (Adler, 2001). Moreover, by shifting the normative concerns of professionals towards bureaucratic efficacy, there is a danger that the patient comes to perceive the norms in which the actions of the professional are embedded as being oriented towards institutional goals rather than considerations of patient-centredness. This is especially the case with concerns of risk, which were described by a number of professional participants as impinging upon effective care:

"Yes. And I think that does make it hard to work with people sometimes in a positive way because you've always at the back of your mind got: 'Well, if this happened will I have done this amount of paperwork, will I be held up?' And I think that does probably impinge on our work a bit really." (*Social worker*)

Such specific notions of risk – understood within the broader concerns of bureaucratic accountability, public perceptions and blame – were unsurprisingly much less explicit within the accounts of service users. Yet the apparently conflicting priorities this social worker (just quoted) acknowledges were frequently referred to. Sometimes this was due to the requirements for professionals to watch out for signs indicating the service user being unwell, but which could be interpreted (in an assertive outreach setting) as intrusive and alienating:

> "It's lots of silly things, you know, like I'll leave a pair of socks on the floor or something and it's 'Oh you can't do that'. 'Have you dusted this week?' And then what about lawful liberty? Whatever happened to lawful liberty? You know, it's my lawful liberty whether I dust my house or not and it's got nothing to do with a social worker." (*Service user 1*)

Thus, attempts at control (not least of 'risk'), as one mode of managing uncertainty and vulnerability, may be seen to be problematic due to the way associated practices destabilise the relationships between professionals and service users, potentially resulting in attitudes of hostility as apparent in the preceding excerpt. The extent to which control is reliant on trust engenders that attempts at achieving control display a tendency to undermine themselves (Brown, 2008a), for 'even when tightly controlled, softer information and informal relationships often underpin formal contracts' (Davies and Mannion, 2000: 251). This is a feature of the trust–control dialectic, whereby the neglect of the social underpinnings of order leads to the demoralisation of healthcare workers as well as a 'de-moralisation' of healthcare work (Brown, 2008a). This latter notion refers to the potential for service users to become treated as risk objects (Castel, 1991) rather than individuals in the midst of professional practice. This phenomenon may occur in spite of the professionals' best intentions, where healthcare practice becomes increasingly instrumental and, thus, blind to the relational. One manifestation of this instrumentality was the suggestion by one professional participant that damage to the reputation of the Trust had implications for the Chief Executive's 'bonus'. The next section explores the mechanisms by which instrumentality at one level of an organisation can spread elsewhere, thus impeding the communicative action in which trust is rooted (Brown, 2008b).

The interrelatedness of trust across different organisational dimensions

Preceding sections have noted the way organisational and managerial tendencies are significant in shaping the interactions of professionals with service users. From a number of perspectives, we can see the interdependent linkages between different levels or dimensions of the organisation in terms of trust – where the prevalence or paucity of trust that exists across one dimension (eg between managers and professionals) has significant ramifications for the extent of trust existing across other dimensions (eg between professionals and service users). This interrelatedness of trust across different dimensions of the organisation has been recognised in some earlier studies (Gilson et al, 2005); though our findings enable a more detailed exposition of some of the complex causality within these interwoven trust dimensions.

One defining concept for understanding the ways in which these different dimensions of trust bear upon one another is *time*. Time, in terms of quantity and quality, is vital to the effective building of trust relations (Davidsen and Reventlow, 2010; Leutwyler and Wallhagen, 2010), whereby the devoting of time by a potential trustee is often decisive in affirming their benevolent motives in the eyes of the truster. Aspects of the literature suggest that time is not necessarily relevant; for example, family doctors are able to build 'swift trust' through skilled communication. However, in our study, a combination of the problematics for trust in mental health services, coupled with the chronicity of care situations and long-term relationships that need to be built between professionals and service users, would seem to make time a highly salient factor for the development of trust:

> "It just seemed like she kind of had some care and concern, which I'm not saying the other guy didn't, but it just seemed like time was *slower* there [respondent's emphasis]. You have to trust them enough to tell them … you know, it's stuff that you feel ashamed about really…. But it really felt like she just kind of put me right up the list for that period of time and that it really didn't matter what else was going on. And this was someone who listened to a lot of my concerns over that period of time." (*Service user 8*)

Time was not only a significant factor contributing towards the positive perceptions of *motives*, but, furthermore, notions of *competence* were also related to time – indirectly through the development of relations. The ability of a professional to deliver effective outcomes for the service user – one important component in order for them to be viewed as competent (and thus trustworthy) – was, in many senses, dependent upon their knowledge of the service user, their awareness of particular needs and their accurate understanding of the service user's condition. Quality relations were typically necessary in order for sufficient length and openness of disclosure by the service user to enable the professional to significantly help the service user. Thus, time is again salient in facilitating outcomes, esteem of competence and, thus, trust.

As well as a necessary 'input' for trust, time can also be seen as a *product* of trusting relationships. Adler (2001), among many, notes that the checking and bureaucracy that trust enables organisations to dispense with thus makes them more efficient. For example, where professionals are trusted more by their managers, there is a reduced bureaucratic burden and more time for trust-building relations through interactions with colleagues and service users. Conversely, low levels of trust between managers and professionals impinge on professional time and, thus, the quality of interactions with other professionals and service users. *Ceteris paribus*, this latter phenomenon is detrimental for trust within these dimensions.

Time, therefore, is significant for trust in a number of senses, not least through the way that it enables the exchange of knowledge. Knowledge, especially that exchanged within effective communication, enables trust to be won (by delivering appropriate and safe outcomes), but, moreover, is an outcome of trust in that trusting relations facilitate learning environments (Sheaff and Pilgrim, 2006) and knowledge exchange (Adler, 2001). In turn, knowledge helps overcome uncertainty, which, as discussed earlier, is also an important feature of the vulnerability experienced by professionals and other actors within mental healthcare contexts.

As with uncertainty, vulnerability both makes trust necessary and is able to be managed through trust. Hence, again, as with time and knowledge, this concept is a key lynchpin in understanding how different dimensions of trust are linked with one another. Limited trust within one dimension renders actors vulnerable, and this impacts on their behaviour within an array of contexts, which bears upon their ability to trust and be trusted across other dimensions. Supervision between more senior and junior professionals is a prime example of a mode by which vulnerability can potentially be managed through a relational-based approach, facilitated by trust:

> "It's like magnetic north ... we're constantly trying to find a position of certainty and it can't be found. So there's a constant ebb and flow of that wish to find certainty about diagnosis or prediction and prognosis – to know exactly when someone's going to hurt themselves or someone else – and trying to live with the fact that you can't predict those things with anything like the degree of certainty that we'd want. So we use supervision; especially group supervision is often taken up with that dynamic." (*Consultant psychologist*)

Supervision is a vital mode of managing vulnerability for both senior and junior professionals. Less experienced professionals need knowledge and guidance to help them manage difficult and unfamiliar circumstances, while the senior professionals need to ensure that effective care is provided, for which they are ultimately responsible. Where an organisational dynamic is relatively bureaucracy-free, as facilitated by managers, supervision can act as a useful basis for exchanging knowledge and enhancing care. This enhances relations between professionals while also undergirding effective outcomes for service users, and, therefore, also enhancing trust relations across the service user–professional dimension too. Yet too many supervision sessions and other meetings may begin to erode time in professional–patient relations:

> "There's lots of supervision – you've already picked up on that!"

> "I'd say client time is probably only a third ... the reason for that is because of travel, meetings and paperwork." (*Social worker*)

Supervision and meetings, though useful, have the potential to become a bureaucratic distraction. They were reported as, at times, having become more to do with checking on professionals' work (a mode of surveillance) as opposed to constructive learning and support – interpreted within the wider characteristics of the modern NHS. Davies and Mannion's (2000) distinction between the facilitating of transactions through trust and/or bureaucratic checking is important here in distinguishing between those supervisory meetings that – facilitated by trust – enable the exchange of useful knowledge and mutual learning, and those meetings that serve the function of hierarchical checking. The latter can be deemed problematic for trust in three key senses. First, the existence of checking indicates a lack of trust in the professional and perpetuates a low-trust inter-professional environment – where the manager/senior colleague may become the visible face of an 'audit culture' (Brown et al, 2011a). Second, it detracts from professionals' time with service users, which, as we have seen, is critical to trust-building. Third, this form of interaction fails to equip the professional – either communicatively or instrumentally – with the necessary support or knowledge to build trust with service users.

Virtuous and vicious circles of trust

In the preceding section, we explored how the levels of trust – or its alternative of checking controls – which exist between managers and professionals have a fundamental impact upon inter-professional trust and, moreover, trust between professionals and service users. The various ways in which *time, knowledge* and *vulnerability* are salient in shaping the creation of trust, while also existing as outcomes of trust, are intrinsic to usefully understanding this interconnectedness. Strongly apparent, albeit somewhat implicit, in the preceding section was the existence of 'circles' of trust – whereby trusting environments seemingly breed effective working relationships that, in turn, enhance trust across various dimensions and so the circle continues. We also came across evidence of more vicious circles where limited levels of trust encouraged more bureaucratic forms of managing vulnerability, with these impinging upon the time and knowledge-sharing within effectual relationships – thus leading to the obstruction of trusting relations in the longer term. As discussed in the preceding section, these obstacles were glaringly evident in terms of the paperwork bureaucracy that was increasingly experienced:

> "Most of the time we should be out there with service users and in the community but increasingly people get very anxious about the fact that their contacts [recording of interactions] need to be updated. And there are so many emails that come through from the Trust about all kinds of nonsense, really.
>
> And it's related to the trustworthiness or untrustworthiness of the whole system, because colleagues' record-keeping is often defensive in my view. So they write reams and reams and reams of contact

> details just in case they ... you know, if they're ever called to account."
> (*Psychologist*)

This kind of record-keeping, as a phenomenon of low trust within the broader NHS mental health system (instituted by policymakers), accordingly comes to significantly colonise professional time, perspectives and work effort. Time, proximity and relationships with clients, and also with other professionals, suffer as a consequence:

> "I think there's an awful lot of pressure around ... particularly in terms of ... how the services are managed centrally and commissioned. But there is a greater requirement for ... I mean people talk about performance targets and we're becoming very orientated towards that ... but that creates a pressure in itself." (*Manager*)

Pressure was apparent for work within this more instrumental NHS to develop goals that are antithetical to trust (Brown, 2008a). Where professional and managerial work became more embedded in the instrumental, in terms of working to bureaucratic checks and targets, the communicative aspects such as relationships, priorities of the patient and sharing of knowledge were harder to uphold (Williamson, 1993). Basic duties to satisfy pressures, such as ensuring risk-minimisation strategies were adhered to, could come to overshadow and distract from spending time getting to know patients as individuals as opposed to risk objects (Castel, 1991). From the perspective of Adler's (2001) model of three sources of trust, familiarity and the sharing of norms and values (the communicative) were being compromised due to the increasing focus on the instrumental – leaving only calculation (the instrumental):

> "Increasing pressure all the time. It's not only the reputation [of the organisation in case of media scrutiny of adverse incidents], it's about lots of things, it's government targets, it's the organisational targets, it's what they call serious untoward incidents. All of this happens all the time and it's becoming even more." (*Psychiatrist*)

These pressures have deleterious effects on the occupational health of professionals. Hence, the impacts of these systemic, bureaucratic pressures upon inter-professional trust were observed as twofold: first, they limit and distract from interactions with colleagues in the short term, inhibiting trust; and, second, the pressures increase staff absences and inhibit the longer-term retention of staff, with both of these features hindering workplace trust-building:

> "If someone is sick a lot or off a lot and not contributing to the team and those types of things and then it starts to feel a little bit uneasy and people start to have splitting and those types of things. They can't trust

that the person is gonna be there all the time, meetings get cancelled or CPA's get cancelled and that's when the trust starts to unbalance and shift the team around; things like that, commitment to work. That's one that comes up here quite a lot." (*Manager*)

Elliot (2004) describes trust as an inoculation against anxiety. In contrast, the heightened pressures and bureaucratic checking experienced by some of the professional informants in our study were evidence of limited levels of trust and – somewhat ironically given the context – led to vicious circles of distrust through staff experiences of poor mental health. Poor retention of quality staff over the longer term, and the inter-professional strains and lack of interaction that results from absences in the shorter term, have detrimental impacts on all dimensions of trust across the organisation:

- Certain service user participants referred to the feeling of being let down by certain care coordinators who had been consistently absent, while the loss of relationship when established care coordinators left the service was also detrimental to outcomes and relations.
- Difficulties in recruiting and retaining quality staff, alongside absences for long-term illness, could also impact upon staff morale and inter-professional relationships. Notable differences existed across the three services within our study with more trusting environments associated with lower absences and better staff retention. This benefited service users as well as staff in the team.
- Where service user outcomes were compromised by staff shortages due to recruitment difficulties and illness, this put greater strain on manager–professional relations. Contact time with service users was vital to effective treatment and accurate risk assessment. Management concerns in these areas required greater levels of bureaucratic checking and this was experienced by professionals as signifying limited trust on the part of managers.

Origins of virtuous and vicious circles

In the preceding two sections, we have referred to three trust dimensions within mental healthcare contexts: service user–professional, inter-professional and professional–manager. While these were the key dimensions explored in our study, it was clear from our data that broader trust-related dimensions are also significant and influential in impacting upon the three dimensions referred to here. The manager quoted earlier in the preceding section refers to broader performance frameworks that foster a particular, pressurised environment. This work environment, following arguments set out in the Introduction, can be considered to be an 'atmosphere' that bears upon trust relations. In the Introduction, we also referred to the expectations and pressures around risk management that exist within late-modern society more generally (Luhmann, 1993) and within mental health contexts more specifically (Pilgrim, 2007). Thus, a chain of contextual 'atmospheres' can be seen to exist, which begins with more general socio-cultural tendencies and the various ways these shape policy. In turn, the resulting policy frameworks and accountability structures impact upon management formats and, thus, working cultures within services.

In the preceding sections, it may seem as though the management approach is decisive in influencing the extent of time, bureaucracy and knowledge exchange, which shape the professionals' (and thus service users') interactive experiences. Yet these managerial formats are themselves embedded within wider constraints set out by the senior management of the local healthcare authority (NHS Partnership Trusts in our research), which, in turn, are oriented by national government policy – in response to (media-influenced) discourses within the public sphere. From this perspective, we can note the interdependence and interaction between the three different dimensions of trust explored earlier, the tendencies for these relations to create virtuous or vicious circles, but we must also clarify that these dynamics are, in many senses, rooted in broader policy frameworks and socio-cultural tendencies that bear decisively on trust relations.

In other work with colleagues (Brown et al, 2011a), we have set out a three-tiered model as a basis for understanding the way management – professional interactions, especially those involving middle and junior managers – are rooted in overarching policy dynamics. This develops a useful linkage between the three-dimensional trust outlined earlier and broader organisational and policy frameworks. Most fundamental is the policy dimension that 'shapes the ways in which junior and middle managers relate to senior managers as well as clinicians, and the tensions or contradictions between these various relationships' (Brown et al, 2011a: 43).

Over time, policy shapes the organisational culture at the local level, with a particular local organisational environment shaping 'the recruiting and development of managers and which may lead to certain types of career background, knowledge frameworks, language and personalities predominating across the managerial workforce' (Brown et al, 2011a: 43). Combined, these two environments – macro-policy and local organisational culture – form a crucial backdrop in which the individual interactions, which are ultimately most decisive for trust, take place. These environments impact on the extent and nature of interactions and the respective goals of the middle managers and professionals, but also provide a whole array of ideal-typical assumptions through which interactions are interpreted. Through this latter mode, it is often the case that middle managers are perceived, in the eyes of professionals, as the embodiment of the policy and organisational initiatives that they are charged with implementing and, in some cases, enforcing.

It would be too simplistic, however, to argue that all trust relations that take place in mental health settings are ultimately a product of policy. That would be to overlook the specific dynamics of trust that were apparent in our data analyses, which distinguish trust in these mental health settings from trust in many other healthcare contexts. Risk-oriented, target-driven, performance-focused policy formats are not in themselves specific to mental healthcare, but, rather, are ubiquitous across the (post–1997) NHS (Harrison and McDonald, 2008). The pressures experienced by staff in our study and the limited nature of trust described are unusual in comparison to other healthcare contexts (as noted in earlier chapters). This suggests some aspects specific to the uncertainty and associated vulnerability that are features of mental health services, especially in the treatment of service users with psychosis diagnoses. Indeed, most professionals and managers recognised the heightened levels of uncertainty and the obstacles faced in developing cooperative relationships with service users (see Seale et al, 2006).

It is important to take this latter analysis one step further. In the preceding chapter, we acknowledged the dangers of merely explaining away our data based on illness alone. As was noted there, mental health problems are grounded in social-environmental factors and, hence, it is these contexts that should also be considered when analysing the specific problems and tensions around trust that our data point towards. As was considered in Chapter Four, following Pilgrim and colleagues (2011), the same social contexts (or fields) that give rise to mental health problems may often also be associated with inculcating forms of *habitus* (dispositions) that are less trusting. It is the tension that exists between the social contexts in which service users are embedded, and which also may tend away from trust, on the one hand, and mental health services, which are embedded within policy formats that tend away from trust, on the other, which would seem to be salient in explaining the trust problems that are apparent within our data and, indeed, the studies of our colleagues (Scrivener, 2010; Maidment et al, 2011).

Figure 5.1: Demands on mental health services – problems for trust

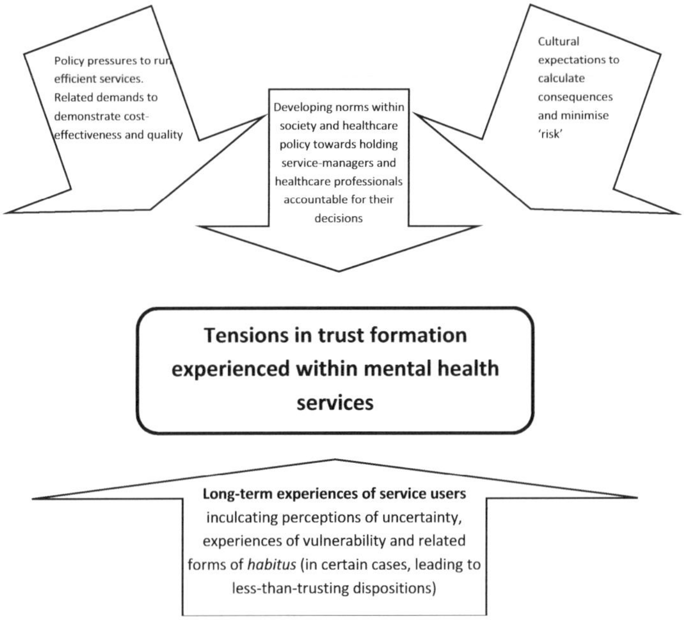

Policy pressures to run efficient services. Related demands to demonstrate cost-effectiveness and quality

Developing norms within society and healthcare policy towards holding service-managers and healthcare professionals accountable for their decisions

Cultural expectations to calculate consequences and minimise 'risk'

Tensions in trust formation experienced within mental health services

Long-term experiences of service users inculcating perceptions of uncertainty, experiences of vulnerability and related forms of *habitus* (in certain cases, leading to less-than-trusting dispositions)

The professionals and middle managers who participated in our research thus carry out their work, which relies on trust, at the intersection of two broader socio-cultural contexts that may often undermine trust. This tension is summed up, in many senses, by the following quote. Here, a social worker refers to the personality traits (or *habitus*) that represent, on the one hand, challenges to attaining effective outcomes and, on the other hand, the culture of risk aversion (driven also by the media) that limits his options in terms of positive risk-taking (entailing trust):

> "And I think that balance is quite hard now. I think that's probably one of the hardest ... and balancing risk, because I think although for some of the people that we work with, who maybe have also personality traits, managing risk becomes even more of a problem there because for them to move forward sometimes you have to take positive risks and I don't think you're always supported enough; not necessarily by members of the [NHS] Trust but by media's perception and what we know will happen when it doesn't go [successfully]." (*Social worker*)

A starting point for potential policy solutions

This double-ended – top-down and bottom-up – understanding of the trust difficulties experienced within mental healthcare settings (see Figure 5.1) is useful as well as instructive regarding the creation of potential solutions to the difficulties faced by managers, professionals and service users. Healthcare policymakers are clearly limited in their ability to engineer social contexts that avoid the development of mental health problems, forms of distrustful *habitus* or personality disorders as referred to in the preceding excerpt. More straightforwardly amenable to change, however, are the policy contexts that create problems from the other side of the interface between the state and those experiencing mental health problems. Adjustments to policy would not, as the model underlines, fully overcome problematic contexts of trust, but would, nonetheless, facilitate relations that were more appropriate for building trust – between managers, professionals and service users.

From the point of view of more overarching policy frameworks, approaches that seek to balance concerns of risk with those around how to most appropriately facilitate and provide resources and, thus, assist access to quality treatment are a clear start in working towards a more trusted mental healthcare system. Recent mental health policy in Scotland has sought to separate concerns over how to manage the risk posed by a small minority of service users from the issues of how best to care for the vast majority (Darjee and Crichton, 2004), and, indeed, this format would seem to have much merit to it, due to this prioritising of care over risk.

It is important that risk and care are not mistaken as being mutually exclusive, yet services that focus upon how best to meet the needs of service users, as understood by these users, will *ceteris paribus* always be more trusted than those that are preoccupied with other concerns (such as risk) that may conflict with service users' interests, and, moreover, which serve to stigmatise these users. At this point, it should be stressed that trust should not be seen as an end in itself, but, rather, as a vital indicator of quality service provision and a useful way of understanding how developments in quality can be facilitated. Purely focusing on how to win the trust of individuals is likely to lapse into people being let down:

> Poor services cannot conjure up 'trust' as a means of masking their deficiencies or erasing the negative previous experiences of their users. Trust, rather, is a useful tool in pointing services towards an essential aspect of quality – and understanding how needs may most adequately be met. (Brown et al, 2009: 456)

As discussed earlier, because of the ways in which trust and control are bound up with one another, attempts to manage vulnerability and uncertainty through control and risk tend to be problematic for trust. Hence, at both the macro-policy and local organisational level, approaches that seek to de-emphasise the bureaucratic mode of holding people accountable for failings will enable better healthcare provision and management of risk through the trust that is facilitated. Crucial here is the development of knowledge within organisations and the relationship of this to trust. As considered earlier in this chapter, organisations that rely relatively less on bureaucratic control and more on trust are often more sophisticated in their capacity for developing and disseminating knowledge (Adler, 2001; Sheaff and Pilgrim, 2006). Knowledge is vital for enhancing outcomes, managing risk, developing professionals and, therefore, delivering quality care and building trust. Where sufficient time for communication and familiarity are developed – within organisations and between the organisation and its users – trust will be won, which, in turn, will augment knowledge-sharing yet further, thus enhancing outcomes (Green et al, 2008).

The preceding paragraphs, and, indeed, the wider arguments presented in this book, are not suggesting that the management of risk and the bureaucratic pursuit of organisational control and accountability are inherently problematic – nor should they be dispensed with. Rather, as we have argued elsewhere (Brown and Calnan, 2010; 2011):

1. there are a range of ways of approaching risk and quality management other than a more top-down approach;
2. notions of trust are useful in considering the adequacy and appropriateness of these frameworks for healthcare governance;
3. concerns around trust are vital for successful governance; and
4. considerations of the relationship between trust and control can provide us with very useful insights into how to better design and manage services at the local level.

Conclusion

This chapter began by emphasising that it is not only mental healthcare service users who face heightened levels of vulnerability and uncertainty, but professionals and managers also deal with a wide range of unknowns, which – within the socio–political contexts of local services that demand high levels of prediction, accuracy and accountability – render these health service workers vulnerable. Not only are the organisational dynamics of a service partially the *source* of vulnerability amidst uncertainty, but, of course, they also shape the responses of professionals within these contexts. These formats of professional action are reproduced as perceived norms of work (amidst vulnerability), shaping and constraining professional conduct through their existence as an 'objective' social reality, while also being created by the actions of professionals and managers who perpetuate these certain norms of behaviour (Berger and Luckmann, 1966). We have argued here that either these modes of coping with vulnerability may tend more towards interpersonal/trust-based solutions, which lead to the refinement of communication and shared understandings within the service, or that professionals and managers tend, instead, towards more bureaucratic/control-oriented solutions, which rationalise the service towards a more goal-focused, instrumental logic of professional behaviour and care-giving.

The analysis of our data, following Habermas (1987), suggests that the goal-oriented rationality of the latter approach has a tendency to neglect the humanness of service users and, therefore, also overlook the salience of relationships, time spent in interactions and familiarity, as well as the concerns of the spaces where these interactions take place. These ultimately undermine the transference of knowledge between service users and professionals, between different professionals, and between professionals and managers. This, in itself, is problematic for risk management and general outcomes. In contrast, the communicative basis of the interpersonal/trust-based approach is likely not only to lead to better-quality interactions, but, furthermore, to enhance the attainment of goals within service provision – through enhanced knowledge exchange.

Alas, the overarching frameworks for accountability within which mental health services are embedded encourage, or rather demand, a more instrumental approach to service provision. We have argued that although the difficulties that exist for building trust within mental health services are innately problematic due to the nature of the social contexts that contribute to illness experiences and corresponding needs, the policy frameworks that drive local organisational responses could do much more to enable the organisational dynamics that build trust. Central to the analysis presented in this chapter is the interrelatedness of different dimensions of trust within services, the way these interwoven patterns of trust seemingly lead to virtuous or vicious circles, and the partial origins of these circles within policy frameworks.

As with related studies (Scrivener, 2010; Maidment et al, 2011), our research found much evidence of many trusting relationships. Yet the analysis around such data points to the way these existed partly in spite of organisational-bureaucratic pressures and policy frameworks – through quality of care, empathy and skilled communication acted out amidst the pressures faced by professionals – as opposed to being facilitated by them. Thus, although a number of accounts that pointed towards the professional-communicative competence and high motivations of staff were useful in explaining this trust, lower levels of trust appeared to exist overall and a number of informants – professionals, managers and service users – referred to trust as distinctly problematic, either currently or in the past.

Accordingly, professionals are very much trusting on the edge, with the difficulties or hindrances they face costing them much – not least in the high levels of work pressures and stress[5] that were reported. Trust, as an 'inoculation' against anxiety (Elliott, 2004), should be valued in its potential utility for enhancing the experiences of not just service users, but also professionals and managers. Critical reflection upon the forms of bureaucratic control used, the bureaucratic burden associated with this, the way knowledge is managed and the extent of time and space that exists for relations and familiarity to be developed will help orient local organisations as to how they may reorganise and manage themselves in order to facilitate trust (for more on the interplay between workplace stress, time and interactions, see Davidsen and Reventlow, 2010); although their capacity to do this and build trust-enabling organisations is ultimately bounded within the parameters laid out within central policy frameworks.

Notes

[1] 'Conduct of conduct' was a term coined by Foucault and is central to many 'governmentality' approaches that are grounded in Foucauldian insights. For a useful introduction to this field, see Burchell and colleagues (1991).

[2] It should be clarified that the 'will to trust' we refer to here can be conceptualised somewhat differently to the 'will to trust' referred to in Chapter Four with regard to service users. Whereas both forms of willingness are embedded within social contexts, the professionals' 'will to trust' seemed to hinge to a degree on a particular 'moral' ideal, that professionals had a duty to trust their patients/service users. Such ideals were less apparent within the accounts of service users and much of the impetus for their 'will to trust' came from seeking to cope as effectively as possible with the vulnerability and uncertainty they faced.

[3] Davies and Mannion (2000) also draw attention to the interwoven-ness and mutual dependency of these two organisational dynamics.

[4] This professional was qualified as both a CPN and a social worker.

[5] One study goes as far as to suggest that an important attribute of mental health professionals is an ability to deal with stress (Schout et al, 2010).

SIX

Trusting on the edge: implications for policy

This final chapter has two main aims. First, to summarise the major themes that emerged from the theoretical and empirical analysis and discuss their implications for furthering the understanding of the nature and salience of trust relations in the context of mental healthcare and beyond. This will involve a summary of the key conclusions that emerge from the different elements of the analysis. The second aim is to consider the policy implications that flow from the empirical findings and the theoretical framework. While policy notions are applied throughout this book and form the very context within which theorisations are developed, this concluding chapter will more explicitly draw out a number of considerations and challenges for policy and practice, based on the findings of the research. More specifically, it will explore theoretical propositions that services organised around concerns of trust will: be more likely to be approached by those in need; enable more complete and open 'disclosure' between service users and professionals (Dew et al, 2007); and facilitate greater levels of cooperation with agreed treatment plans. Key questions for further research will also be identified where relevant.

Overview of key themes

The underlying purpose of our research was to explore the nature of trust in this context of heightened vulnerability and uncertainty. Hence, the focus here is on the clinical setting of the provision of mental health services where there is not only uncertainty about diagnostic labels (many of which are still associated with both felt and enacted stigma) and treatment outcomes, but where the nature of the trusting relationship may be integral to the modes of treatment and, therefore, fundamental to therapeutic outcomes. Certainly, trust is not something immediately identifiable, but, rather, tends to be taken for granted and routinised. Thus, its existence may not come to the fore until it is challenged and where there is at least the threat of a breakdown in trust between service users and clinicians, or between clinicians and their managers.

A study of trust in action, therefore, needed to focus on situations where trust is fragile, such as in the context of mental healthcare, which was believed to be a 'low-trust' setting (Helene Hem et al, 2008; Pilgrim et al, 2011). This is a relatively neglected topic for research (Laugharne and Priebe, 2006; Brown et al, 2009) so we explored how trust in its different forms (more or less conditional, distrust or positive mistrust) might influence (intermediate) outcomes – primarily for service users, but also for professionals and managers. Our research in other areas (Calnan and Rowe, 2008; Brown et al, 2011b) had indicated that trust relations across one dimension – for example, between managers and professionals – had ramifications for other dimensions – such as inter-professional trust and professional–service user trust (as explored in Chapter Five).

Our analysis was informed by these perspectives alongside a range of other key themes, which included: risk and control; the construction of knowledge frameworks as a basis for making inferences about the future; and time. The first of these, risk and control, is not only a significant theme in the trust literature, but has also been a defining feature of recent English health service policy, and so will be addressed again in the final section that specifically examines policy implications.

Examining the construction of knowledge by participants, through the application of interpretive frameworks, was useful in demonstrating how trust relations can be developed even in the problematic context of mental health services (as seen in Chapter Two). The generally negative portrayal of the competencies and intentions of mental health services and psychiatry within the public sphere was seen as often having been accompanied by a range of negative consequences and outcomes for the service users we interviewed.

And, yet, it was shown both theoretically and empirically that there are a number of ways in which these apparent barriers to trust could be overcome. The possibilities for trust in spite of apparently good reasons why service users would not trust were seen as being rooted in the nature of trust as an active, constructed and pragmatic endeavour by which knowledge is inferred through past experiences. Drawing on Schutzian phenomenology (Schutz, 1972), we argued that three different forms of experience – mediated, public-direct and private-interactive – were invoked within this inferential process, although private experiences are the most concrete and, therefore, relevant for trust (see Chapter Two).

Another key theme of the analysis was the salience of the concept of time, which emerged in a number of different contexts. Time had been a vital factor in our previous analyses of trust through the way that the devoting of time by busy professionals was inferred as demonstrating their benevolence and care (eg Brown et al, 2011b). Time was also a fundamental component of the analysis within the current study, partly due to the way that the process of trust is inherently involved with linking experiences and knowledge from the past to considerations and expectations regarding the future.

In another sense, the feature of familiarity is one key mode by which time is influential for trust. The manner by which knowledge is able to be inferred and applied in contexts where trust may be necessary is significantly influenced by the degree of familiarity with which the truster perceives the setting and personnel (Luhmann, 1979). Time is clearly crucial to continuity of care and length of relationships and the extent to which these were influential (or not) for trust. The time (quantity and quality) needed for the effective development of trust relations emerged as highly significant for informants, and, indeed, the concept of time was seen as vital to understandings of associations between trust relations across different dimensions – adding much to understandings of linkages within Gilson and colleagues' (2005) model; for example, the way in which workplace trust impacts on professional behaviour and attitudes and, therefore, on service user trust.

Economic perspectives consider trust as a lubricating force (Williamson, 1993), freeing up employees and resources – especially time – through diminished checking. In contrast, the bureaucratic system described by the professional and managerial informants in our study engendered significant time spent on paperwork and meetings, which distracted from service user interactions. Also evident was a corresponding defensiveness. Professionals were acutely aware of the conduct of their conduct (Warner, 2006), with this instrumentally oriented action at odds with the communicative focus of trust-building.

The concept of time was also central to the analysis of the relationship between trust and choice. The significance of different time dimensions within choice, and, indeed, dependence as a result of certain choices (or limitations of choice), offered a more detailed understanding of the ways in which choice, dependence and, thus, trust impact on one another within social processes. Understanding trust as a process (Khodyakov, 2007), rather than a one-off decision, was accordingly seen as significant in incorporating and describing the agency of trusters – even amidst conditions of dependence – as well as offering a more accurate conception of trust within dynamic social relations. Trust is decisive to understanding certain 'decision moments', which invariably are vital to healthcare outcomes, yet the expectations that are central to trust are not momentary phenomena in themselves. This ongoing process of trust and its dynamic development within certain relationships is especially apparent within the chronic treatment contexts of mental health services.

The experiences of professionals and managers

At a more substantive level, the analysis threw some light on a number of salient but under-researched questions. The first of these concerns the perspective of the clinician and the manager in trust relations. The empirical literature about trust relations in healthcare in general (for a review, see Calnan and Rowe, 2008) has been dominated, probably for good reasons, by the experience and perspectives of the users and/or the public. This was evident in this study in that high levels of uncertainty and vulnerability were experienced by service users, and the *chronic* experiences of mental health service users mean that trust relations take place within a distinct format – with the development of deeper long-term relations vital given the chronicity, effects of stigma and negative past experiences (eg of involuntary detention).

Yet there also appear to be uncertainties and vulnerabilities that the clinician has to face and manage, such as where there is a risk of making a diagnostic error or risking a professional reputation by treating patients or service users[1] with ambiguous symptoms in a certain way. Given the amount of unverifiable, descriptive information that a clinician must rely on from a given patient, a clinician is presented with a situation in which his or her trust in the service user could be called into question as they may or may not believe the symptoms being presented to them. Patients' reported symptoms may confound common understandings and this may cause clinicians to doubt the patient's testimony rather than the prevailing scientific evidence. This could be especially true in contexts where a patient might be perceived as exaggerating their claims, which may alter how they are ultimately treated. Pilgrim et al (2011:27) expand on these considerations by arguing that lay-people might not be trusted by clinicians to act in their own interests because of a perception of poor decision-making due to lack of knowledge (competence-related trust) and lack of care for their health (intention-related trust), due to 'passivity, nihilism, fatalism and fecklessness and at worst because they use help-seeking and illness presentation for manipulative reasons' (for a study that acknowledges obstacles to cooperation from the perspective of psychiatrists, see also Seale et al, 2006).

A related issue is self-trust or intra-personal trust, which Pilgrim and colleagues (2011) refer to as 'confidence in ourselves'. Self-trust may be particularly salient for less-experienced clinicians who have clinical discretion but feel vulnerable as they do not have the confidence in their own competence, may be less willing to take risks and will, thus, tend to follow protocols and rely on tests that may lead to a lack of personalised care, which may have consequences for patient trust. Further research is needed in this area and, in particular, might pursue the way in which service contexts inculcate certain dispositions towards a lack of self-trust or confidence among practitioners, or, alternatively, where treatment contexts may foster a *habitus* of overconfidence or exaggerated self-trust – both can be problematic and potentially damaging for patient experiences. Levels of self-trust are likely to vary around profession (in terms of status and power), experience, local service culture and management formats, but also the socio-cultural backgrounds from which professionals are most typically recruited.

The evidence presented in this study clearly suggests that professionals and managers in mental healthcare settings deal with a wide range of uncertainties that may make self-trust less likely. Within the socio-political contexts of local services that demand high levels of prediction, accuracy and accountability coupled to a media fascination with risk and mental illness and a fashion for blaming individual experts and services, healthcare workers are rendered vulnerable and prone to stress and anxiety. Not only are the organisational dynamics of a service partially the source of vulnerability and uncertainty, but they also shape the responses of professionals and managers within these contexts (see Chapter Five and Figure 6.1).

We have argued that these responses may tend either more towards interpersonal/ trust-based solutions, which lead to the refinement of communication within the service, or that professionals and managers tend, instead, towards more bureaucratic/control-oriented solutions, which rationalise the service towards a more goal-focused, instrumental logic of professional behaviour and care-giving.

In this latter sense, professionals may potentially become like *street-level bureaucrats* (Taylor and Kelly, 2006) – those practitioners in the public sector on the 'front line' (directly dealing with patients or service users) who use bureaucratic procedures and interpret rules to pursue their tasks in the easiest way possible. Such instrumentalisation of professional work (see also Eraut, 1994) ultimately undermines the development of knowledge due to a stifling of reflection, but also impedes the transference of knowledge between service users and professionals, between different professionals, and between professionals and managers. Both these consequences are problematic for risk management and general outcomes.

Figure 6.1: A model of factors that bear on manager–professional trust

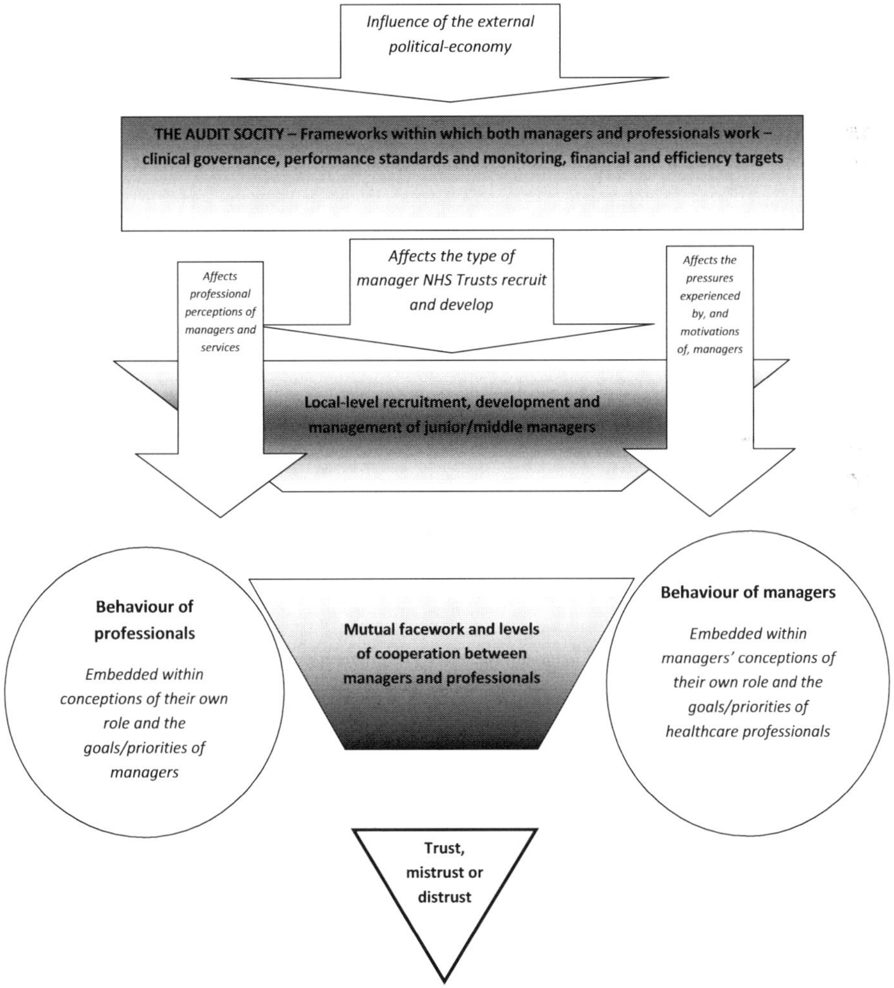

This discussion leads on to the second question that this study provides some insight into – the relationship between the different levels of trust relations, and how system-level trust relations might shape interpersonal relations or vice versa. The analysis has shown the primacy of facework for users, which goes some way to explaining why trust in healthcare systems may be less salient than trust in clinicians (Calnan and Rowe, 2008). Gilson and colleagues (2005) highlight the need for more nuanced understandings of the connections between different dimensions of trust in healthcare provision, the implications for worker performance and the corresponding impact on patient–provider trust. Central to our analysis has been the interrelatedness of different dimensions of trust within services and also the way these interwoven patterns of trust seemingly lead to virtuous and vicious circles (see Chapter Five).

As has been emphasised throughout the book and particularly in Chapter Five, professional participants in this study experienced especially elevated levels of uncertainty in this domain of healthcare. Accordingly, this places their work exceedingly at odds with the demands for the 'calculability of consequences' (Weber, 1978: 351) that are a feature of modern, bureaucratic healthcare systems (Harrison, 2009). Unable to meet these demands, professionals experienced significant vulnerability and, in a number of cases, anxiety. Central to the relationship between levels of workplace trust and patient–provider trust are the interactions between vulnerability and uncertainty, time and communicative action. Reactions of vulnerability amidst uncertainty at one level (eg managerial or professional) accordingly impact upon the depth of relations at other levels in terms of familiarity, shared norms and values, and awareness of interests (Adler, 2001). The policy pressures that currently exist, in terms of efficiency and risk assessment, impede trust relations across the services – directly and indirectly making the recruitment and retention of quality staff problematic.

Our research, however, did find evidence of many trusting relationships, suggesting that clinicians and practitioners have some latitude to develop strategies to balance risk assessment and its associated bureaucratic procedures with a more personalised and empathetic approach. The empirical analysis points to the way these strategies existed in spite of organisational bureaucracy and policy, as opposed to being facilitated by them. Thus, although a number of accounts that pointed towards the professional-communicative competence and high motivations of staff were useful in explaining this trust (Schout et al, 2010), lower levels of trust appeared to exist overall and a number of informants – professionals, managers and service users – referred to trust as distinctly problematic. Much critical reflection is necessary, on the part of senior managers in particular, as to how services may foster more trusting environments that, in turn, will facilitate the trust-building work of professionals with service users; although, as we noted in Chapter Five, the capacity for senior managers (and, indeed, middle and junior managers) to adopt such an approach is in many ways limited by existing policy frameworks and corresponding preoccupations with risk.

Policy implications: rediscovering trust

This penultimate section addresses the policy implications that emerge from the theoretical and empirical analysis. The basic argument is, given the analysis previously reviewed, that policy should shift towards an emphasis on enhancing trust relations and away from the current emphasis on risk, although it is recognised that such a shift will not solve all of the many difficulties currently associated with the provision of mental health services in England.

The policy narrative about the NHS, particularly the NHS in England, over the last decade or more has been characterised by the introduction of principles from the new public management aimed at improving accountability, efficiency and quality of care (Calnan and Rowe, 2008). Such policies have involved the use of performance targets, audit and monitoring, and risk management. The increasing priority is claimed now to be based on assessing institutional risk rather than meeting patient needs (Kemshall, 2002). One reason for the introduction of the externally regulated accountability frameworks that appear to constrain clinical discretion and actions was the consequences of a series of media–amplified scandals over medical competence in the 1990s. Clearly, it was perceived within certain circles that clinicians could not be trusted to regulate one another to ensure that they were competent enough and working in the interests of their patients.

The impact of these policies on professional practices have been well documented, particularly the tensions between health service managers and clinicians (Brown et al, 2011a). It is suggested that the distraction of the professionals' need to satisfy stipulations and accountability frameworks diverts their attention away from the patients' interests. The greater the extent to which this is the case, the more the audit society (Power, 1997) 'robs actors of the meaning of their own actions' (Habermas, 1987: 302) and, therefore, comes to be resented by the professional (Brown and Calnan, 2011). This is especially the case where 'what gets measured has to be done', but where the measurable, biomedical indicators of quality are blind to a more holistic notion of patient care (Brown, 2008a).

Such concerns are highly pertinent in the field of psychiatry where outcomes and quality might be best understood more qualitatively. Certainly, the governance and accountability frameworks associated with the new public management techniques would seem to generate cultures of low trust 'as trust has an inverse relationship with demands for explicit accountability; high trust relations result in limited demands for explicit accountability and low trust relations produce increased demands for explicit evidence of the same' (Calnan and Rowe, 2008: 31). Market-mechanism modes of governance (which recent English governments have returned to) are similarly associated with cultures of low trust because of a lack of trust in professional and public service norms and values (Sheaff and Pilgrim, 2006).

This emphasis on risk in English health policy is clearly reflected in mental health policy where it has been a defining principle. Jones (1972) characterises recent mental health policy as oscillating between legal and medical approaches, that is, between risk and need, and as neglecting more *social* approaches that put an emphasis on human relations. Our findings suggest that not only does this risk preoccupation represent an obstacle to meeting need, but it may also be self-defeating in the effective management of risk – as visible in the vicious circle of trust we have described in Chapter Five. This can be contrasted with an alternative model whereby services focused on winning/earning the trust of service users would meet health and social needs more effectively and, moreover, be better placed to curtail risk – through the creation of virtuous circles of trust, as illustrated earlier.

Primarily, the utility of trust has been understood through its facilitating of access/engagement, disclosure and cooperation with services. As is evident from the data (and emphasised through the 'circle' analogy), these three factors – access, disclosure and cooperation – are very much interwoven. For example, continuing engagement and clearer communication regarding medication side effects/ problems, lifestyle changes or substance misuse will enable more appropriate care-giving and prescribing. This would enhance the meeting of needs (through improved cooperation) while also serving to attenuate the risk attached to lapses in medication cooperation and substance misuse where these arise (Swartz et al, 1998).

Thus, trust exhibits the qualities of a 'solvent of clinical risk' (Wilkinson, 2004: 94), while concurrently enabling action to meet need amidst vulnerability and uncertainty. For example, one study (Thogersen et al, 2010) exploring the views on, and perceptions of, coercion of users in Danish assertive community teams showed that users reported: a lack of influence in the treatment process and a poor alliance with case managers; not being recognised as autonomous individuals; and perceiving staff as overly intruding upon their privacy. These shaped experiences of coercion, which echo the experiences described by our respondents involved with assertive outreach (service user and professionals). A collaborative and mutually trusting relationship, the commitment, persistence and availability of staff, and the recognition of the need for social support and help with everyday activities, were most important for counteracting such experiences (Thogersen et al, 2010). These authors concluded that developing mental health practices that enhance the formation of a therapeutic relationship with service users will minimise circumstances that induce perceptions of coercion.

One possible danger of carrying out a study to explore the nature and salience of trust in relationships between users and clinicians is that researchers will tend to overemphasise its importance. However, although our findings did suggest that constructive outcomes are still possible in the absence of trust (see Box 2.2), trust was described as highly pertinent by the service users giving accounts of more positive outcomes. In either case, the relevance of 'the social' – in achieving mutual understanding or, at the least, agreements to differ – was highly effectual. Thus, it would seem that the comparative neglect of the social channel, as apparent within Jones' (1972, 1993) accounts, has hindered mental health services, and a rebalancing towards the social and away from the procedural is necessary. This is not to argue that services should dispense with risk management, but, rather, that the social and that which builds trust should be esteemed more highly – and protected when it is threatened by the procedural. Service users often referred to their relationships with (and trust of) professionals being undermined by practices that were seemingly a result of procedural necessity. Meanwhile, all care coordinators described the bureaucratic burden that limited the time they could spend with service users.

More theoretically, this tension can be understood through a phenomenon that has been referred to as the 'trust–control dialectic' (see Brown, 2008a; following Gallivan and Depledge, 2003), whereby concerted attempts to achieve control through procedure ultimately serve to undermine trust (social channels) and correspondingly control (see Chapter Five). As Gellner (1988: 143) argues, 'it is effective government which destroys trust' and, correspondingly, the therapeutic relationship on which the provision of quality care and the accurate assessment of risk depends (MIND, 2004). Risk, as a control-oriented calculative approach to uncertainty, can be seen as contrasting sharply with trusting approaches – the latter adheres to a person-centred approach while the former 'trusts' in technologies of control. Moves towards bureaucratic and calculative control can also be seen as antithetical to trust (Gellner, 1988) in that these technocratic approaches are rooted in a lack of trust in individuals (Brown and Calnan, 2010) – for example, service users and professionals – eroding the role of norms on which trust is based.

Flowing from such an understanding is the requirement for services to find a new balance between trust and control, one more disposed towards the former than is currently the case. This balance should protect against the dark side of trust, for example, the dangers of exploitation in an asymmetrical relationship, while avoiding the negative consequences of checking – for example, defensive practice. Trade-offs between dealing with risk through control or trust are best considered in terms of how the two may most appropriately be balanced, rather than an either/or scenario (Davies and Mannion, 2000). Chapter Five, following Möllering (2005), noted how trust and control are very much dependent upon one another. The paradox of relaxing risk proceduralism in order to manage risk (through trust) more effectively makes it a less likely policy avenue to be pursued, and yet it is necessary if trust is to enable the improvements in access, disclosure and medication cooperation that our findings point towards.

The Care Programme Approach (CPA) may be usefully designed to bring existing information together to enable a more adequate assessment of risk, and to avoid people 'slipping through the net' of services. Yet, while this knowledge may be more consistently recorded, this bureaucratic element must be balanced with the goal of relationship-building with service users to provide them with sufficient grounds for assuming that services will continue to act in their best interests – thus encouraging them to disclose more openly. Otherwise, services will only be accumulating superficial or distinctly selective accounts from service users, which will help little with improving outcomes (in terms of need or risk).

How, then, can professionals and practitioners be given the discretion to provide high-quality, personalised care for mental health service users? One alternative approach, which has been outlined elsewhere (Brown and Calnan, 2011), is for local clinical leads to oversee and coordinate a peer-monitoring system by which all relevant professionals work together to develop agreed criteria to assess performance and refine standards that are transparent and visible, but not imposed. Hence, trust and cooperation become the central bases for assessing performance and quality

Paths for future research

This research has focused on trust relationships in the context of the provision of care for users who are in the midst of serious mental health problems where, as has been shown, trust relations are fragile. This might be explained by the nature of the users' problems in combination with the recent clinical and organisational approaches to mental healthcare. Our previous research into trust relations was carried out in clinical settings primarily involving the care and treatment of somatic conditions such as diabetes and those requiring hip surgery (Calnan and Rowe, 2008) and gynaecological oncology (Brown, 2009a; Brown et al, 2011b). In these clinical contexts, overall levels of trust were relatively high, although trust was conditional and needed to be earned. Further research might need, therefore, to explore clinical contexts that bridge the physical and psychological, such as chronic fatigue syndrome and fibromyalgia where symptoms are diffuse and non-specific, where it is difficult to find supportive clinical evidence from tests, and where diagnoses are problematic and contested, thus leading to the use of such labels as 'its all in the head' (Wainwright et al, 2006). In these contexts, maintaining trust relations might be problematic both for users and clinicians.

One advantage of focusing on clinical settings where trust levels are relatively low is that it should be easier to provide insights into how trust might be developed and built up. Evidence from previous empirical research (Calnan and Rowe, 2008) suggests that trust between patients and clinicians depends on factors associated with relationships rather than characteristics of the patient. This evidence suggests that trust can be built if patient views are respected and taken seriously and information is openly shared with patients. However, as well as clinicians' interpersonal skills, their technical competence is important for the development of trust. Yet, a recent review of interventions for improving patients' trust in doctors concluded that no published intervention has yet been effective in improving it (McKinstry et al, 2008).

The importance of relations in building trust was clearly borne out in this current study, which showed that the demonstration of care and technical competence, through quality communication and respectful relationships, combined with the effective and consistent meeting of needs, was fundamental. Both of these facets require sufficient resource provision in order to attract skilled staff and afford them sufficient time across their caseload to build relationships, provide useful care and demonstrate reliability.

There will continue to be patients who will be less likely to trust, or who will hold mistrustful attitudes towards services. This is due to a complex range of factors including the nature of illness conditions, previous histories of being let down and/or compelled by services, and more general dispositional tendencies (rooted in social contexts). Yet the apparent utility of trust as outlined here (see also Leutwyler and Wallhagen, 2010) warrants further research into how services (as organisations) and individual professionals can more adequately build trust as it appears to be fundamental to understanding human resource issues as well as analysing their impact, especially on the quality of care experienced by service users and the development of the supportive learning/working environments that are required for this (Davidsen and Reventlow, 2010; Leutwyler and Wallhagen, 2010).

Theoretically, we have argued based on the data analysed in this study that communicative action (through familiarity, shared norms and quality relationships) facilitates positive outcomes at the instrumental level (eg professional learning; more accurate knowledge of the needs of service users), yet instrumental action in itself (management checking; professional bureaucratic adherence; service users' non-cooperation with care) does not improve outcomes and stifles communication. Research is necessary across a broader range of mental health services (and healthcare settings more generally) to test and refine the theoretical approaches outlined here, especially across a larger and more ethnically diverse population. For example, studies have shown (Keating and Robertson, 2004) that the relationships between black communities and the mental health services in England are tense and that there are 'circles of fear' that lead to poorer treatment of black communities. Sources of fear included perceptions of mental health services, attitudes to mental illness and diagnosis, and experiences of hospital care. The impact of fear included limited trust, limited engagement and delayed help-seeking behaviour. The authors concluded that these fears obstruct the interactions between these communities and mental health services and affect help-seeking behaviour adversely – leading to restrictive and punitive interventions (Keating and Robertson, 2004).

We have argued that the overarching frameworks for accountability within which mental health services are embedded, at least within the NHS in England, encourage or, rather, demand a more instrumental approach to service provision. Although the difficulties that exist for building trust within mental health services may be innately problematic due to the nature of the illness and corresponding needs, the policy frameworks that drive local organisational responses could do much more to enable the organisational dynamics that build trust. In order to explore the relative influence of policy frameworks, further comparative research needs to be carried out in different healthcare systems where health policy narratives, more specifically those relating to mental health policy, have been shaped or dominated by principles other than risk: for example, by medical or social approaches to treatment and care, where the emphasis is on rehabilitation, cooperation and trust.

There is also the related but increasingly salient issue, at least in the English NHS, of how mental healthcare is funded and whether trust relationships at the different levels are influenced by the extent to which care is funded and/or provided by the public, private or third sector or a mixture of all three. It might be argued that the more the service is driven by financial as opposed to clinical imperatives (ie the need to make a profit), the lower the levels of trust are likely to be. Evidence from countries such as Australia, which has a more mixed, pluralistic system of healthcare, suggests that a form of trust (symbolic trust) is crucial to the public's decisions to subscribe to private health insurance (Natalier and Willis, 2008). However, survey evidence suggests that the relationship is not straightforward, as higher levels of trust were found in private as opposed to public hospitals, but greater trust in Medicare rather than private health insurance (Hardie and Critchley, 2008).

Finally, what of the implications of trust for important healthcare processes and outcomes? The evidence presented here suggests that trust relations have consequences for access to mental health services, disclosure and adherence, which we understand as intermediate outcomes. However, it is still not clear whether particular forms and levels of trust between users and their mental healthcare providers have benefits for patients and service users in terms of improved clinical and mental health status outcomes, and, if so, how these effects might be mediated. Also, as has been suggested, the trust that service users place in healthcare providers may be more or less active and informed, with potentially different consequences for the kinds of choices and contributions that patients are able and willing to make in relation to their healthcare, and, thus, to their healthcare outcomes.

These and other possible causal pathways between trust and health, including the possibility that trust has direct therapeutic benefits and is key to the placebo or healing effect, need to be examined. Some of the potential dangers of blind or assumed trust have been identified and, although in certain contexts of mental healthcare services lower levels of trust may be both understandable and appropriate, key questions remain over what levels and types of trust contribute to positive mental health outcomes and effective healthcare delivery. Further questions exist as to whether positive outcomes for the organisation are compatible with positive outcomes for service users and clinicians. In terms of trust relations among and between professionals and managers within mental healthcare organisations, there are still important questions to be investigated about the relationships between trust and performance and the factors that are effectual in mediating these relationships.

Note
[1] This chapter, in its generalised perspective, refers to patients *and* service users, but, for the sake of brevity, will just to refer to patients or service users from here onwards.

Appendix

Methods

A phenomenological approach as a 'sensitising' framework

The analytical frameworks developed in this book were all useful in formulating an array of empirical markers pertaining to the existence, nature and/or limits of trust. More particularly, we were especially attentive to various modes by which trust was linked across different dimensions of healthcare services, partially building on an initial framework set out by Gilson and colleagues (2005). Trust has been portrayed in this study as dynamic and contingent. Accordingly, changes in trust levels over time and features associated with this (those that were held to lead to changes in trust, as well as features associated with the resultant effects of changes in trust) received particular attention within the analysis.

As articulated in Chapter One, trust – as a construction of expectations – is very much dependent on how attitudes and behaviours are *interpreted* and then inferred to indicate intentions of action – regarding trustees' interests and embeddedness within normative structures (Möllering, 2005). These features of trust as a process of building knowledge from an array of experiential sources indicated the utility of a phenomenological approach as a 'sensitising' framework (Hammersley and Atkinson, 2007), which informed both the format of interviews and the coding of data (see more on phenomenology as an approach to trust in Chapter One).

In this way, the difficulty of identifying and coding the potentially nebulous concept of trust was overcome. A focus on the interpretive experiences of actors and the way these were drawn upon when constructing future expectations was recognised as especially salient when coding understandings of trust – as an ongoing, embodied, conditional and negotiated process of sense-making and expectation construction (Smith and Osborn, 2003). When analysing the data, the informants' use of ideal-types (Schutz, 1972) was also apparent and noted – for example, generalised views of the quality of mental health services, the motives of psychiatrists or the likely concordance of certain service users. This ideal-typical knowledge formed important building blocks when constructing future expectations (Brown, 2009a).

Design

The dynamics of different trust relations were explored through a single case study involving informal interviews with service users, professionals and managers (*n* = 23) working in three services designed to meet the needs of people experiencing psychosis – all within one NHS Trust (local health authority) in Southern England. These three contrasting services (mini cases) – an early intervention team, an

assertive outreach team and a more standard community mental health team –
were purposively selected in order to explore the relevance and nature of trust
across different team and care contexts.

Sampling and participants

The manager, clinical lead (two consultant psychiatrists and a consultant
psychologist) and two to three other professionals in each of the three settings,
including at least one community psychiatric nurse and social worker per team,
were purposively sampled participants. The majority of the professional participants
had considerable experience (mean duration working in mental health services
= 16.1 years; SD = 10.6). To add a further dimension to our data collection, we
also included a mental healthcare chaplain among our interview participants.

Recruitment of service users in each context (eight users and one carer targeted
in each setting) proved much more problematic. Inclusion criteria were all users in
each service aged 18 and over, while only those who were experiencing a more
acute phase of their illness were excluded. A number of different recruitment
strategies were adopted beginning with a letter and pre-paid envelope sent via
professionals, followed by a similar approach but with a financial (gift voucher)
incentive and, finally, attempts were made to identify participants through snowball
sampling. Letters of invitation were sent out to 158 participants leading to eight
service users being interviewed. Carers were to be recruited via users, with one
carer being interviewed.

Despite these difficulties, the service user participants reflected a diverse range
of backgrounds and experiences (mean duration of contact with services = 15.9
years; SD = 12.4), spanning gender (four in each), a broad age range (from 25
to 67), education levels (from leaving school at 16 to postgraduate study and
increments in between) and economic activity (out-of-work; voluntary work;
paid part-time work; retired). Two were in the earlier stages of their illnesses and
had limited experience with the mental health services (less than two years), but
the remainder had at least 10 years' experience. Efforts to recruit an ethnically
diverse range of participants were not successful.

This latter limitation, alongside the broader recruitment problems, might be seen
as indicative of the vulnerability of the population we were trying to access, the
practical and ethical difficulties associated with this (Smith, 2008), and the limited
capacity to adopt a more flexible recruitment strategy due to research governance
bureaucracy. The difficulties could, furthermore, be interpreted as indicating that
the trust problems our data point towards may in fact be much more profound.
Several studies on variations in levels of trust in the US show that lower levels
of trust in doctors were associated with African-Americans compared to white
Americans (Calnan and Rowe, 2008). Such disparities may be particularly relevant
for UK mental health services given perceptions within certain ethnic minority
communities of differential attitudes and treatment (Appleby, 2008).

Data collection

The professional and manager interviews were thematic (typically 30 minutes to one hour), addressing issues of working with and relating to clients, how positive outcomes were pursued, and the general challenges of the job (including managing risk). As with all the interviews, although trust was the central focus of the research, direct questions regarding the concept were sequenced towards the end of the interviews in order to examine the relevance of trust as it emerged naturally within participants' accounts. Questions then sought to clarify the relevance (or extraneousness) of trust for participants.

The service user and carer interviews followed a longer (50 minutes to one and three quarter hours), more narrative format commencing from first illness experience, with emerging themes revisited for further clarification towards the end of the interview, along with key questions that had not emerged initially within the narrative. Again, initial probing related to positive and negative aspects of contact with services, relations with key professionals and psychiatrists, and only latterly around the relevance of trust for their experiences and outcomes. The study attained local NHS ethics committee and research governance clearance. Interviews took place between January and November 2010.

Method of analysis

The interview recordings were re-listened to, transcribed and coded. N-Vivo was used to facilitate analysis. Double-coding and critical discussions around the coding process were carried out to assist with the interpretive rigour of the analysis. Basic coding was carried out after each interview in order for emergent themes to be fed back into future interviews. Latterly, inductive thematic analysis was applied incorporating three stages of coding – open, axial and selective (Neuman, 1997). 'Open' refers to seeking a very broad range of potentially relevant factors, partially influenced by the sensitising framework outlined earlier, which directed special attention to the construction of assumptions and meanings within the lifeworlds of participants (Smith and Osborn, 2003). 'Axial' coding involved the assembling of these initial codes into a more coherent framework, using the method of constant comparison and, within this process, highlighting certain recurring and salient concepts and processes. These more developed understandings were then further refined and nuanced through 'selective' application across cases, paying particular attention to deviant cases and the implications of these for the development of overall understandings.

References

Adler, P. (2001) 'Market, hierarchy, and trust: the knowledge economy and the future of capitalism'. *Organization Science* 12(2): 215–34.

Adorno, T. and Horkheimer, M. (1973) *Dialectic of Enlightenment*. London: Allen Lane.

Akerlof, G. and Shiller, R. (2009) *Animal Spirits: How Human Psychology Drives the Economy, and Why It Matters for Global Capitalism*. Princeton, NJ: Princeton University Press.

Alaszewski, A. (2002) 'The impact of the Bristol Royal Infirmary disaster and inquiry on public services in the UK'. *Journal of Interprofessional Care* 16(4): 371–8.

Alaszewski, A. and Brown, P. (2007) 'Risk, uncertainty and knowledge'. *Health, Risk and Society* 9(1): 1–10.

Alaszewski, A. and Brown, P. (2012) *Making Health Policy: A Critical Introduction*. Cambridge: Polity.

Alaszewski, A. and Burgess, A. (2007) 'Risk, time and reason'. *Health, Risk and Society* 9(4): 349–58.

Appleby, J. and Alvarez-Rosete, A. (2003) 'The NHS: keeping up with public expectations?'. In: K. Park, J. Curtice, K. Thomson, L. Jarvis, and C. Bromley. (eds) *British Social Attitudes: Continuity and Change over Two Decades*. London: Sage, pp 29–44.

Appleby, L. (2008) 'Services for ethnic minorities: a question of trust'. *Psychiatric Bulletin* 32(11): 401–2.

Ashraf, N., Bohnet, I. and Piankov, N. (2003) 'Is trust a bad investment?'. John F. Kennedy School of Government Harvard University Faculty Research Working Papers Series.

Baas, D., van't Wout, M., Aleman, A. and Kahn, R. (2008) 'Social judgement in clinically stable patients with schizophrenia and healthy relatives: behavioural evidence of social brain dysfunction'. *Psychological Medicine* 38(5): 747–54.

Barbalet, J. (2009) 'A characterisation of trust, and its consequences'. *Theory and Society* 38(4): 367–82.

Barber, B. (1983) *The Logic and Limits of Trust*. New Brunswick: Rutgers University Press.

Bauman, Z. (2000) *Liquid Modernity*. Cambridge: Polity

Beahrs, J. (1986) *Limits of Scientific Psychiatry: The Role of Uncertainty in Mental Health*. New York: Brunner/Mazel.

Beck, U. (1992) *Risk Society: Towards a New Modernity*. London: Sage.

Berger, P. and Luckmann, T. (1966) *The Social Construction of Reality*. London: Penguin.

Best, J. (1999) *Random Violence: How We Talk about New Crimes and New Victims*. Berkeley: University of California Press.

Blumer, H. (1969) *Symbolic Interactionism: Perspective and Method*. Englewood Cliffs, NJ: Prentice Hall.

Bourdieu, P. and Wacquant, L. (1992) *An Invitation to Reflexive Sociology*. Chicago, IL: University of Chicago Press.

Britten, N. (1998) 'Psychiatry, stigma and resistance'. *British Medical Journal* 317: 963.

Brown, N. and Webster, A. (2004) *New Medical Technologies and Society: Reordering Life*. Cambridge: Polity.

Brown, P. (1987) 'Diagnostic conflict and contradiction in psychiatry'. *Journal of Health and Social Behaviour* 28(1): 37–50.

Brown, P. (2006) 'Risk versus need in revising the 1983 Mental Health Act: conflicting claims, muddled policy'. *Health, Risk and Society* 8(4): 343–58.

Brown, P. (2008a) 'Legitimacy chasing its own tail: theorising clinical governance through a critique of instrumental reason'. *Social Theory and Health* 6: 184–99.

Brown, P. (2008b) 'Trusting in the new NHS: instrumental *versus* communicative action'. *Sociology of Health and Illness* 30(3): 349–63.

Brown, P. (2008c) *The Impact of Clinical Governance and the Audit Culture on Patient Trust: The Opportunity Cost of Instrumental Rationality*. PhD Thesis, University of Kent, Canterbury.

Brown, P. (2009a) 'The phenomenology of trust: a Schutzian analysis of the social construction of knowledge by gynae-oncology patients'. *Health, Risk and Society* 11(5): 391–407.

Brown, P. (2009b) 'Beyond reason? The limitations of rationality as a tautological and asocial concept'. Paper presented at the conference 'Varieties of Risk Research: Exploring and Expanding Boundaries within Academia and Beyond', Kings College, London, 5 June.

Brown, P. (2011) 'The dark side of hope and trust: constructed expectations and the value-for-money regulation of new medicines'. *Health Sociology Review* 20(4): 407–19.

Brown, P. and Calnan, M. (2010) 'The risks of managing uncertainty: the limitations of governance and choice, and the potential for trust'. *Social Policy and Society* 9(1): 13–24.

Brown, P. and Calnan, M. (2011) 'The civilizing process of trust: developing quality mechanisms which are local, professional-led and thus legitimate'. *Social Policy and Administration* 45(1): 19–34.

Brown, P. and Calnan, M. (forthcoming) 'NICE technology appraisals: the potential for bias in the midst of uncertainty'. *Medicine, Healthcare and Philosophy*. DOI: 10.1007/s11019-011-9376-2

Brown, P. and Flores, R. (2011) 'Making normative structures visible: the British National Health Service and the hospice movement as signifiers of compassion and hope'. *Acta Sociologica* 54(1): 61–75.

Brown, P., Calnan, M., Scrivener, A. and Szmukler, G. (2009) 'Trust in mental health services: a neglected concept'. *Journal of Mental Health* 18(5): 449–58.

Brown, P., Alaszewski, A., Pilgrim, D. and Calnan, M. (2011a) 'The quality of interaction between managers and professionals: a question of trust'. *Public Money and Management* 31(1): 43–50.

Brown, P., Alaszewski, A., Swift, T. and Nordin, A. (2011b) 'Actions speak louder than words: the embodiment of trust by professionals in gynae-oncology'. *Sociology of Health and Illness* 33(2): 280–95.

Brownlie, J., Greene, A. and Howson, A. (2008) *Researching Trust and Health*. London: Routledge.

Brubaker, R. (1984) *The Limits of Rationality: An Essay on the Social and Moral Thought of Max Weber*. London: Allen and Unwin.

Burawoy, M. (1998) 'The extended case method'. *Sociological Theory* 16(1): 4–33.

Burchell, G., Gordon, C. and Miller, P. (1991) *The Foucault Effect: Studies in Governmentality*. Hemel Hempstead: Harvester Wheatsheaf.

Burns, T. and Priebe, S. (1999) 'Mental healthcare failure in England: myth and reality'. *British Journal of Psychiatry* 174: 191–2.

Calnan, M. and Rowe, R. (2008) *Trust Matters in Healthcare*. Buckingham: Open University Press.

Calnan, M. and Sanford, E. (2004) 'Public trust in health care: the system or the doctor'. *Quality and Safety in Health Care* 13: 92–7.

Calnan, M., Rowe, R. and Entwistle, V. (2006) 'Trust relations in health care: an agenda for future research'. *Journal of Health Organisation and Management* 20(5): 477–84.

Castel, R. (1991) 'From dangerousness to risk'. In: G. Burchell, C. Gordon and P. Miller (eds) *The Foucault Effect – Studies in Governmentality*. Hemel Hempstead: Harvester Wheatsheaf, pp 281–98.

Cherrington Hughes, E. (1994) 'Mistakes at work'. In: L. Coser (ed) *Everett C. Hughes – On Work, Race and the Sociological Imagination*. Chicago: University of Chicago, pp 79–89.

Cohen, S. (2002) *Folk Devils and Moral Panics*. London: Routledge.

Coleman, J. (1983) 'Recontracting, trustworthiness and the stability of vote exchanges'. *Public Choice* 40: 89–94.

Cooper, D. (1967) *Psychiatry and Anti-Psychiatry*. London: Tavistock.

Cornwell, J. (1985) *Hard-Earned Lives: Accounts of Health and Illness from East London*. London: Tavistock.

Corrigan, P. and Watson, A. (2002) 'The paradox of self-stigma and mental illness'. *Clinical Psychology* 9(1): 35–53.

Couture, S., Penn, D., Addington, S., Woods, S. and Perkins, D. (2008) 'Assessment of social judgments and complex mental states in the early phases of psychosis'. *Schizophrenia Research* 100(1): 237–41.

Crossley, N. (1998) 'R. D. Laing and the British anti-psychiatry movement: a socio-historical analysis'. *Social Science and Medicine* 47(7): 877–89.

Danermark, B., Ekström, M., Jakobsen, L. and Karlsson, J. (2002) *Explaining Society: Critical Realism and the Social Sciences*. Abingdon: Taylor and Francis.

Darjee, R. and Crichton, J. (2004) 'New mental health legislation'. *British Medical Journal* 329: 634.

Davidsen, A.S. and Reventlow, S. (2010) '"It takes some time to get into the rhythm – and to slow the flow of thought": a qualitative study about experience of time and narrative in psychological interventions in general practice'. *Health: an Interdisciplinary Journal for the Social Study of Health, Illness and Medicine* 14(4): 348–68.

Davies, H. and Mannion, R. (2000) 'Clinical governance: striking a balance between checking and trusting'. In: P. Smith (ed) *Reforming Markets in Health Care: An Economic Perspective*. Buckingham: Open University Press, pp 246–67.

Department of Health (1995) *Building Bridges. A Guide to Arrangements for Interagency Working for the Care and Protection of Seriously Mentally Ill People*. London: HMSO.

Department of Health (2000) *The NHS Plan: A Plan for Investment, A Plan For Reform*. London: TSO.

Department of Health (2007) *The Mental Health Act, 2007*. London: HMSO.

Dew, K., Morgan, S., Dowell, A., McLeod, D., Bushnell, J. and Collings, S. (2007) '"It puts things out of your control": fear of consequences as a barrier to patient disclosure of mental health issues to general practitioners'. *Sociology of Health and Illness* 29(7): 1059–74.

Dibben, M. and Davies, H. (2004) 'Trustworthy doctors in confidence building systems'. *Quality and Safety in Health Care* 13: 88–9.

Dibben, M. and Lean, M. (2003) 'Achieving compliance in chronic illness management: illustrations of trust relationships between physicians and nutrition clinic patients'. *Health, Risk and Society* 5: 241–8.

Douglas, M. (1992) *Risk and Blame: Essays in Cultural Theory*. London: Routledge.

Dunn, J. (1993) 'Trust'. In: R. Goodin and P. Pettit (eds) *A Companion to Contemporary Philosophy*. Oxford: Blackwell, pp 638–44.

Eastman, N. (1996) 'Inquiry into homicides by psychiatric patients: systematic audit should replace mandatory inquiries'. *British Medical Journal* 313: 1069.

Elliott, A. (2002) 'Beck's sociology of risk: a critical assessment'. *Sociology* 36(2): 293–315.

Elliott, A. (2004) *Subject to Ourselves: Social Theory, Psychoanalysis and Postmodernity* (2nd edn). Boulder, CO: Paradigm.

Entwistle, V., Watt, I., Bradbury, R. and Pehl, L. (1996) 'Media coverage of the Child-B case'. *British Medical Journal* 312: 1587–91.

Eraut, M. (1994) *Developing Professional Knowledge and Competence*. London: Routledge.

Flynn, R. (2002) 'Clinical governance and governmentality'. *Health, Risk and Society* 4(2): 155–70.

Freedman, D. (2002) 'Clinical governance – bridging management and clinical approaches to quality in the UK'. *Clinica Chimica Acta* 319: 133–41.

Fugelli, P. (2001) 'Trust – in general practice'. *British Journal of General Practice* 51: 575–9.

Furedi, F. (2002) *Culture of Fear: Risk Taking and the Morality of Low Expectation*. London: Cassell.

Gallivan, M. and Depledge, G. (2003) 'Trust, control and the role of interorganizational systems in electronic partnerships'. *Information Systems Journal* 13(2): 159–90.

Gellner, E. (1988) 'Trust, cohesion, and the social order'. In: D. Gambetta (ed) *Trust: Making and Breaking Cooperative Relations*. Oxford: Blackwell, pp 142–57.

Giddens, A. (1990) *The Consequences of Modernity*. Cambridge: Polity.

Giddens, A. (1991) *Modernity and Self-Identity: Self and Society in the Late Modern Age*. Cambridge: Polity.

Giddens, A. (1994) 'Living in a post-traditional society'. In: U. Beck, A. Giddens and S. Lash (eds) *Reflexive Modernisation: Politics, Tradition and Aesthetics in the Modern Social Order*. Cambridge: Polity.

Gigerenzer, G. (2007) *Gut Feelings: the Intelligence of the Unconscious*. New York: Viking.

Gigerenzer, G. and Brighton, H. (2009) 'Homo Heuristicus: why biased minds make better inferences'. *Topics in Cognitive Science* 1(1): 107–43.

Gigerenzer, G. and Todd, P. (1999) *Simple Heuristics That Make Us Smart*. Oxford: Oxford University Press.

Gilson, L., Palmer, N. and Schneider, H. (2005) 'Trust and health worker performance: exploring a conceptual framework using South African evidence'. *Social Science and Medicine* 61: 1418–29.

Goffman, E. (1963) *Stigma: Notes on the Management of Spoiled Identity*. New York: Simon and Schuster.

Gray, B. (1993) *The Profit Motive and Patient Care: The Changing Accountability of Doctors and Hospitals*. Cambridge, MA: Harvard University Press.

Gray, J. (2009a) 'We simply do not know'. *London Review of Books* 31(22): 13–14.

Gray, J. (2009b) 'The original modernizers'. In: J. Gray (ed) *Gray's Anatomy – Selected Writings*. London: Allen Lane.

Green, C., Polen, M., Janoff, S., Castleton, D., Wisdom, J., Vuckovic, N., Perrin, N., Paulson, R. and Oken, S. (2008) 'Understanding how clinician–patient relationships and relational continuity of care affect recovery from serious mental illness: STARS study results'. *Psychiatric Rehabilitation Journal* 32(1): 9–22.

Habermas, J. (1971) *Toward a Rational Society: Student Protest, Science and Politics*. London: Heinemann.

Habermas, J. (1976) *Legitimation Crisis*. Boston, MA: Beacon.

Habermas, J. (1984) *Theory of Communicative Action. Volume One: Reason and the Rationalisation of Society*. Boston, MA: Beacon.

Habermas, J. (1987) *Theory of Communicative Action. Volume Two: Lifeworld and System: a Critique of Functionalist Reason*. Cambridge: Polity.

Haddow, G. and Cunningham-Burley, S. (2008) 'Tokens of trust or token trust? The case of population genetic data collections'. In: J. Brownlie, A. Greene, and A. Howson (eds) *Researching Trust and Health*. London: Routledge, pp 152–73.

Hall, M., Dugan, E., Zheng, B. and Mishra, A. (2001) 'Trust in physicians and medical institutions: what is it, can it be measured, and does it matter?'. *Milbank Quarterly* 79: 613–39.

Hallam, A. (2002) 'Media influences on mental health policy: long-term effects of the Clunis and Silcock cases'. *International Review of Psychiatry* 14(1): 26–33.

Hammersley, M. and Atkinson, P. (2007) *Ethnography: Principles in Practice.* London: Routledge.

Hardey, M. (1999) 'Doctor in the house: the Internet as a source of lay health knowledge and the challenge to expertise'. *Sociology of Health and Illness* 21: 820–35.

Hardie, E.A. and Critchley, C.R. (2008) 'Public perceptions of Australia's doctors, hospitals and health care systems'. *Med J Australia* 189(4): 210–14.

Hardin, R. (1992) 'The street-level epistemology of trust'. *Analyse & Kritik* 14: S152–S176.

Harrison, S. (2009) 'Co-optation, commodification and the medical model: governing UK medicine since 1991'. *Public Administration* 87(2): 184–97.

Harrison, S. and McDonald, R. (2008) *The Politics of Healthcare in Britain.* London: Sage.

Harrison, S. and Smith, C. (2004) 'Trust and moral motivation: redundant resources in healthcare'. *Policy and Politics* 32(3): 371–86.

Helene Hem, M., Heggen, K. and Ruyter, K. (2008) 'Creating trust in an acute psychiatric ward'. *Nursing Ethics* 15(6): 777–88.

Hirschey, M. and Nofsinger, J. (2009) *Investments: Analysis and Behavior.* New York: McGraw–Hill.

Hobbes, T. (1968 [1651]) *Leviathan.* London: Penguin.

Hochschild, A. (1979) 'Emotion work, feeling rules and social structure'. *American Journal of Sociology* 85(3): 551–75.

Hood, C. (2005) 'Trust relations in the new NHS: theoretical and methodological challenges'. Paper presented at the conference 'Taking Stock of Trust', London School of Economics and Political Science, London, 12 December.

Huang, B. and Priebe, S. (2003) 'Media coverage of mental healthcare in the UK, USA and Australia'. *Psychiatric Bulletin* 27: 331–3.

Inglis, T. (2010) 'Sociological forensics: illuminating the whole from the particular'. *Sociology* 44(3): 507–22.

Japp, K. and Kusche, I. (2008) 'Systems theory and risk'. In: J. Zinn (ed) *Social Theories of Risk and Uncertainty.* Oxford: Blackwell, pp 76–105.

Joint Committee (2005) 'Joint Committee on the Draft Mental Health Bill – First Report'. Available at: http://www.publications.parliament.uk/pa/jt200405/jtselect/jtment/79/7902.htm (accessed 10 July 2005).

Jones, I.R., Leontowitsch, M. and Higgs, P. (2010) 'The experience of retirement in second modernity: generational habitus amongst retired senior managers'. *Sociology* 44(1): 103–20.

Jones, K. (1972) *A History of the Mental Health Services.* London: Routledge & Kegan-Paul.

Jones, K. (1993) *Asylums and After: A Revised History of the Mental Health Services, from the Early Eighteenth Century to the 1990s.* London: Athlone.

Keating, F. and Robertson, D. (2004) 'Fear, black people and mental illness: a vicious circle?'. *Health & Social Care in the Community* 12(5): 439–47.

Kemshall, H. (2002) *Risk, Social Policy and Welfare*. Buckingham: Open University.

Kewell, B. (2006) 'Language games and tragedy: the Bristol Royal Infirmary disaster revisited'. *Health, Risk and Society* 8(4): 359–77.

Keynes, J.M. (1936) *The General Theory of Employment, Interest and Money*. London: Macmillan.

Khodyakov, D. (2007) 'Trust as a process: a three-dimensional approach'. *Sociology* 41(1): 115–132.

Kierkegaard, S. (1957) *Concept of Dread*. Princeton, NJ: Princeton University Press.

Kirk, S. and Kutchens, H. (1992) *The Selling of DSM: The Rhetoric of Science in Psychiatry*. New Brunswick: Transaction.

Knight, F. (1921) *Risk, Uncertainty and Profit*. Boston, MA: Houghton Mifflin.

Lam, A. (2000) 'Tacit knowledge, organizational learning and societal institutions – an integrated framework'. *Organization Studies* 21: 487–513.

Langan, J. (2010) 'Challenging assumptions about risk factors and the role of screening for violence risk in the field of mental health'. *Health, Risk and Society* 12(2): 85–100.

Langlois, R. and Cosgel, M. (1993) 'Frank Knight on risk, uncertainty and the firm: a new interpretation'. *Economic Inquiry* 31: 456–65.

Laugharne, R. and Priebe, S. (2006) 'Trust, choice and power in mental health: a literature review'. *Social Psychiatry &Psychiatric Epidemiology* 41: 843–52.

Lee-Treweek, G. (2002) 'Trust in complementary medicine: the case of cranial osteopathy'. *Sociological Review* 50(1): 48–68.

Leutwyler, H. and Wallhagen, M. (2010) ,Understanding physical health of older adults with schizophrenia building and eroding trust'. *Journal of Gerontological Nursing* 36(5): 38–45.

Lindblom, C. (1959) 'The science of "muddling through"'. *Public Administration Review* 19: 79–88.

Link, B., Cullen, F., Struening, E. and Shrout, P. (1989) 'A modified labeling theory approach to mental disorders: an empirical assessment'. *American Sociological Review* 54(3): 400–23.

Lomranz, J. and Benyamini, Y. (2009) 'Aintegration in Management of Personal and Work-Organizational Conflicting Situations in Modern Society'. Paper presented at the SCARR conference 'Managing the Social Impacts of Change from a Risk Perspective', jointly organised with CASS, Beijing Normal University, ESRC, RCUK, University of Kent, at the Beijing Normal University, Beijing, China 15–17 April.

Luhmann, N. (1979) *Trust and Power*. Chichester: Wiley.

Luhmann, N. (1988) 'Familiarity, confidence, trust: problems and alternatives'. In: D. Gambetta (ed) *Trust: Making and Breaking Cooperative Relations*. Oxford: Basil Blackwell, pp 94–108.

Luhmann, N. (1993) *Risk: A Sociological Theory*. New York: de Gruyter.

Maidment, I., Brown, P. and Calnan, M. (2011) 'An exploratory study of the role of trust in medication management within mental health services'. *International Journal of Clinical Pharmacy* 33(4): 614–20.

McKinstry, B., Ashcroft, R., Car, J., Freeman, G.K. and Sheikh, A. (2008) 'Interventions for improving patients' trust in doctors and groups of doctors'. Cochrane Database of Systematic Reviews, Issue 3, Art No: CD004134.

Mead, G.H. (1962) *Mind, Self and Society*. Chicago: University of Chicago Press.

Mechanic, D. (1996) 'The impact of managed care on patients' trust in medical care and their physicians'. *JAMA* 275(21): 1693–7.

Merleau-Ponty, M. (1968) *The Visible and the Invisible*. Evanston: Northwestern University Press.

Meyer, S. and Ward, P.R. (2009) 'Reworking the sociology of trust: making a semantic distinction between trust and dependence'. Refereed conference paper for TASA Conference, 'The Future of Sociology', 1–4 December, Canberra, Australia, http://www.tasa.org.au/conferences/conferencepapers09/papers/Meyer,%20Samantha.pdf. ISBN of conference proceedings: 978-0-646-52501-3.

MIND (2004). Submission to the Joint Committee on the Draft Mental Health Bill: Summary. Accessed 15 November 2006 from: http://www.mind.org.uk/NR/rdonlyres/1BC535C1-3CB3-4BBF-81F2-09543AA3E668/0/SummaryofMindsubmissiontoJointCommittee.pdf

Misztal, B. (1996) *Trust in Modern Societies*. Cambridge: Polity Press.

Möllering, G. (2001) 'The nature of trust: from Georg Simmel to a theory of expectation, interpretation and suspension. *Sociology* 35(2): 403–20.

Möllering, G. (2005) 'The trust/control duality: an integrative perspective on positive expectations of others'. *International Sociology* 20(3): 283–305.

Möllering, G. (2006) *Trust: Reason, Routine and Reflexivity*. Oxford: Elsevier.

Moncrieff, J. (2010) 'Psychiatric diagnosis as a political device'. *Social Theory and Health* 8(4): 370–82.

MORI (2004) *In Search of Lost Trust*. London: MORI.

Murray, R. (2008) 'The fall and rise again of social factors in psychosis'. Conference paper presented at Mediterranean Maudsley Forum, Palermo, Italy, 24 September.

Mythen, G. and Walklate, S. (2006) *Beyond the Risk Society: Critical Reflections on Risk and Human Security*. Buckingham: Open University Press.

Natalier, K. and Willis, K. (2008) 'Taking responsibility or averting risk? A socio-cultural approach to risk and trust in private health insurance decisions'. *Health, Risk and Society* 10(4): 399–411.

Nettleton, S., Burrows, R. and O'Malley, L. (2005) 'The mundane realities of the everyday lay use of the internet for health, and their consequences for media convergence'. *Sociology of Health and Illness* 27(7): 972–92.

Nettleton, S., Burrows, R. and Watt, I. (2008) 'Regulating medical bodies? The consequences of the "modernisation" of the NHS and the disembodiment of clinical knowledge'. *Sociology of Health and Illness* 30(3): 333–48.

Neuman, W. (1997) *Social Research Methods: Qualitative and Quantitative Approaches*, Boston: Allyn and Bacon.

Newman, J. and Vidler, E. (2006) 'Discriminating customers, responsible patients, empowered users: consumerism and the modernisation of health care'. *Journal of Social Policy* 35(2): 193–209.

Nussbaum, M. (2001) *Upheavals of Thought: The Intelligence of Emotions.* Cambridge: Cambridge University Press.

O'Neill, J. (1995) *The Poverty of Post-Modernity.* London: Routledge.

O'Neill, O. (2002) *Autonomy and Trust in Bioethics.* Cambridge: Cambridge University Press.

Parr, H. and Davidson, J. (2008) '"Virtual trust": online emotional intimacies in mental health support'. In: J. Brownlie, A. Greene, and A. Howson (eds) *Researching Trust and Health.* London: Routledge, pp 33–53.

Petit, P. (1995) 'The cunning of trust'. *Philosophy and Public Affairs* 24(3): 202–25.

Piippo, J. and Aaltonen, J. (2008) 'Mental health care: trust and mistrust in different caring contexts'. *Journal of Clinical Nursing* 17(21): 2867–74.

Pilgrim, D. (2007) 'New "mental health" legislation for England and Wales: some aspects of consensus and conflict'. *Journal of Social Policy* 36(1): 79–95.

Pilgrim, D. and Benthall, R. (1999) 'The medicalisation of misery: a critical realist analysis of the concept of depression'. *Journal of Mental Health* 8(3): 261–74.

Pilgrim, D. and Rogers, A. (2009) 'Survival and its discontents'. *Sociology of Health and Illness* 31(7): 947–61.

Pilgrim, D., Tomasini, F. and Vassilev, I. (2011) *Examining Trust in Healthcare: A Multidisciplinary Perspective.* London: Palgrave.

Pixley, J. (2004) *Emotions and Finance: Distrust and Uncertainty in Global Markets.* Cambridge: Cambridge University Press.

Porter, R. (2001) *The Enlightenment.* Basingstoke: Palgrave Macmillan.

Power, M. (1997) *The Audit Society: Rituals of Verification.* Oxford: Oxford University Press.

Putnam, R. (2000) *Bowling Alone: The Collapse and Revival of American Community.* New York: Simon and Schuster.

Riordan, S. and Humphreys, M. (2007) 'Patient perceptions of medium secure care'. *Medicine, Science and the Law* 47(1): 20–6.

Rogers, A. and Pilgrim, D. (1991) '"Pulling down churches": accounting for the mental health users' movement'. *Sociology of Health and Illness* 13(2) 129–48.

Rothstein, H. (2006) 'The institutional origins of risk: a new agenda for risk research'. *Health, Risk and Society* 8(3): 215–21.

Salter, B. (1999) 'Change in the governance of medicine: the politics of self-regulation'. *Policy and Politics* 27(2): 143–58.

Sartre, J.-P. (1962 [1939]) *A Sketch for a Theory of the Emotions.* London: Methuen.

Scambler, G. and Britten, N. (2001) 'System, lifeworld and doctor–patient interaction: issues of trust in a changing world'. In: G. Scambler (ed) *Habermas, Critical Theory and Health.* London: Routledge, pp 45–64.

Schön, D. (1983) *The Reflective Practitioner: How Professionals Think in Action.* New York: Basic Books.

Schout, G., De Jong, G. and Zeelen, J. (2010) 'Establishing contact and gaining trust: an exploratory study of care avoidance'. *Journal of Advanced Nursing* 66(2): 324–33.

Schrank, B., Stanghellini, G. and Slade, M. (2008) 'Hope in psychiatry: a review of the literature'. *Acta Psychiatrica Scandinavica* 118(6): 421–33.

Schutz, A. (1972) *The Phenomenology of the Social World*. London: Heinemann.

Scrivener, A. (2010) 'Trust in the prescriber of antipsychotic medication in young adult clients of an early intervention service'. Unpublished DClinPsych thesis.

Seale, C. (2003) 'Health and the media: an overview'. *Sociology of Health and Illness* 25(6): 513–31.

Seale, C., Chaplin, R., Lelliott, P. and Quirk, A. (2006) 'Sharing decisions in consultations involving anti-psychotic medication: a qualitative study of psychiatrists' experiences'. *Social Science and Medicine* 62(11): 2861–73.

Sennett, R. (2008) *The Craftsman*. London: Allen Lane.

Sheaff, R. and Pilgrim, D. (2006) 'Can learning organizations survive in the newer NHS?'. *Implementation Science* 1(27). DOI:10.1186/1748-5908-1-27.

Shilling, C. and Mellor, P. (2007) 'Cultures of embodied experience: technology, religion and body pedagogics'. *The Sociological Review* 55(3): 531–49.

Siegrist, M. (2011) 'Lay people's risk perception – The importance of trust and confidence'. Keynote address to the 'Risk, Uncertainty and Policy' Mid-term Conference of Research Network 22 of the European Sociological Association, Östersund, Sweden, 23 March.

Simmel, G. (1950) *The Sociology of Georg Simmel*. New York: Free Press.

Simmel, G. (1990) *The Philosophy of Money* (2nd edn). London: Routledge.

Simon, H.A. (1976) *Administrative Behavior* (3rd edn). New York: Free Press.

Simon, H. (1982) *Models of Bounded Rationality: Behavioral Economics and Business Organization*. Cambridge, MA: The MIT Press.

Smith, L. (2008) 'How ethical is ethical research? Recruiting marginalized, vulnerable groups into health services research'. *Journal of Advanced Nursing* 62(2): 248–57.

Smith, R. (1998) 'All changed, all changed utterly: British medicine will be transformed by the Bristol case'. *British Medical Journal* 316: 1917–18.

Smith, J. and Osborn, M. (2003) 'Interpretative phenomenological analysis'. In: G. Breakwell (ed) *Doing Social Psychology Research*. Oxford: Blackwell.

Solbjør, M. (2008) '"You have to have trust in those pictures": a perspective on women's experiences of mammography screening'. In: J. Brownlie, A. Greene and A. Howson (eds) *Researching Trust and Health*. London: Routledge, pp 54–71.

Solbjør, M., Skolbekken, J.-A., Sætnan, A.R., Hagen, A.I. and Forsmo, S. (2010) 'Mammography screening and trust: the case of interval breast cancer'. Paper presented to the conference 'BSA Medical Sociology', Durham University, 2 September.

Sterne, J. (2003) 'Bureaumentality'. In: J. Bratich, J. Packer and C. McCarthy (eds) *Foucault, Cultural Studies and Governmentality*. Albany, NY: State University of New York Press.

Swartz, M., Swanson, J., Hiday, V., Borum, R. et al (1998) 'Violence and severe mental illness: the effects of substance abuse and nonadherence to medication'. *American Journal of Psychiatry* 155: 226–31.

Szmukler, G. (2001) 'A new mental health (and public protection) act'. *British Medical Journal* 322: 2–3.

Szmukler, G. (2003) 'Risk assessment: numbers and values'. *The Psychiatrist* 27: 205–7.

Sztompka, P. (1999) *Trust: A Sociological Theory*. Cambridge: Cambridge University Press.

Taylor, I. and Kelly, J. (2006) 'Professionals, discretion and public sector reform in the UK: revisiting Lipsky'. *International Journal of Public Sector Management* 19(7): 629–42.

Taylor-Gooby, P. (2000) 'Risk and welfare'. In: P. Taylor-Gooby (ed) *Risk, Trust and Welfare*. Basingstoke: Macmillan, pp 1–18.

Taylor-Gooby, P. (2008) *Reframing Social Citizenship*. Oxford: Oxford University Press.

Thaler, R. and Sunstein, C. (2008) *Nudge: Improving Decisions about Health, Wealth and Happiness*. London: Penguin.

Thogersen, M., Morthorst, B. and Nordentoft, M. (2010) 'Perceptions of coercion in the community: a qualitative study of patients in a Danish assertive community treatment team'. *Psychiatric Quarterly* 81(1): 35–47.

Thorne, S. and Robinson, C. (1989) 'Guarded alliance: healthcare relationships in chronic illness'. *Journal of Nursing Scholarship* 21(3): 153–7.

Tiedens, L. and Linton, S. (2001) 'Judgment under emotional certainty and uncertainty: the effects of specific emotions on information processing'. *Journal of Personality & Social Psychology* 81: 973–88.

Titmuss, R. (2004) 'Choice and the welfare state'. In: A. Oakley and J. Barker (eds) *Private Complaints and Public Health: Richard Titmuss on the National Health Service*. Bristol: Policy Press, pp 167–74.

Tversky, A. and Kahneman, D. (1974) 'Judgement under uncertainty: heuristics and biases'. *Science* 185: 1127–31.

Vaitkus, S. (1990) 'The crisis as a bankruptcy of trust: the fiduciary attitude, human nature and ethical science'. *International Sociology* 5(3): 287–98.

Vaitkus, S. (1991) *How Is Society Possible: Intersubjectivity and the Fiduciary Attitude as Problems of the Social Group in Mead, Guwitsch and Schutz*. London: Kluwer Academic Publishers.

Wade, C., Chao, M., Kronenberg, F., Cushman, L. and Kalmuss, D. (2008) 'Medical pluralism among American women: results of a national survey'. *Journal of Women's Health* 17(5): 829–40.

Wainwright, D., Calnan, M., O'Neill, C., Winterbottom, A. and Watkins, C. (2006) 'When pain in the arm is "all in the head": the management of medically unexplained suffering in primary care'. *Health, Risk and Society* 8(1): 71-88.

Warner, J. (2006) 'Inquiry reports as active texts and their function in relation to professional practice in mental health'. *Health Risk and Society* 8(3): 223–37.

Waugh, E. (1945) *Brideshead Revisited: The Sacred and Profane Memories of Captain Charles Ryder*. London: Chapman and Hall.

Weber, M. (1968) *Economy and Society* (vol 1). New York: Bedminster.

Weber, M. (1975 [1904]) *Roscher and Knies: the Logical Problems of Historical Economics*. New York, NY: Free Press.

Weber, M. (1978) 'The development of bureaucracy and its relation to law'. In: W. Runciman (ed) *Weber: Selections in Translation*. Cambridge: Cambridge University Press, pp 341–56.

Wilkinson, I. (2001) *Anxiety in a Risk Society*. London: Routledge.

Wilkinson, I. (2010) *Risk, Vulnerability and Everyday Life*. London: Routledge.

Wilkinson, J. (2004) 'The politics of risk and trust in mental health'. *Critical Quarterly* 46: 82–102.

Williamson, O. (1975) *Markets and Hierarchies: Analysis and Antitrust Implications*. New York, NY: Free Press.

Williamson, O. (1993) 'Calculativeness, trust and economic organization'. *Journal of Law and Economics* 36: 453–86.

Young, J.E., Klosko, J. and Weisshar, M.E. (2003) *Schema Therapy: a Practitioner's Guide*. New York, NY: Guilford.

Zinn, J. (2008a) 'Heading into the unknown: everyday strategies for managing risk and uncertainty'. *Health, Risk and Society* 10(5): 439–50.

Zinn, J. (ed) (2008b) *Social Theories of Risk and Uncertainty: An Introduction*. Oxford: Blackwell

Index

Note: Page numbers in *italics* refer to figures. Page numbers followed by the letter *n*, e.g. 103*n*, refer to footnotes.

Printed and bound by CPI Group (UK) Ltd, Croydon, CR0 4YY

17/04/2025

14658860-0001